The Illustrated Herbal Handbook for Everyone

Juliette de Baïracli Levy is a pioneer in the field of herbal medicine and the natural rearing of animals. She has proved over many years that her treatments and diets are safe and effective. A botanist, practical herbalist, soil doctor, and anthologist of gypsy lore, she was born in Manchester of Turkish parentage and now lives in Greece. Her books have been translated into many languages and she is consulted constantly by leading herbalists from all over the world.

THE ILLUSTRATED HERBAL HANDBOOK FOR EVERYONE

Juliette de Baïracli Levy

illustrated by Heather Wood

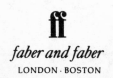

faber and faber

LONDON · BOSTON

First published in 1974
by Faber and Faber Limited
3 Queen Square London WC1N 3AU

Reprinted in 1975 and 1977
Second, revised edition published in
Faber Paperbacks, 1982
Revised with corrections 1991

Printed in Great Britain by
Cox & Wyman Ltd Reading Berkshire

Juliette de Baïracli Levy is hereby identified as author of this work
in accordance with Section 77 of the Copyright, Designs and Patents Act
1988

A CIP record for this book is available from the British Library

ISBN 0-571-16099-9

2 4 6 8 10 9 7 5 3

To
SIR ALBERT HOWARD,
LIND AF HAGEBY, and RIAH KASPI,
who helped forward my herbal work

Important Note for Readers in Great Britain

Since this book was written, the natural habitat of many wild plants has disappeared and some herbs have become rare in the wild because of building developments, intensive farming, and other pressures on land use.

In an effort to prevent these rare plants from extinction, the Wildlife and Countryside Act 1981 and its Variation of Schedule Order 1988 make it an offence for any unauthorized person to pick, uproot, destroy or offer for sale almost a hundred wild plants in Great Britain.

It is also an offence for an unauthorized person to *uproot any wild plant*, whether or not it is on the protected list.

The author strongly advises readers to grow their own herbs or obtain dried herbs from health food shops.

The Wildlife and Countryside Act 1981 and the Wildlife and Countryside Act (Variation of Schedule) Order 1988 can be obtained through HMSO bookshops. Alternatively, a list of the fully protected plant species can be obtained from the Department of the Environment, Tollgate House, Houlton Street, Bristol, BS2 9DJ.

Readers in countries other than Great Britain should check local regulations before gathering flowers in the wild.

Contents

Illustrations

11

ILLUSTRATIONS

1

Introductory

Herbal medicine is man's rightful medicine: the powers of herbs cannot be denied. From the days of the early cavemen to the present time, when human beings are soaring to the moon, people have used herbs to promote and safeguard health and to heal disease. Herbs have also been used very successfully for healing the ills of those animals which man has domesticated. Some of us have special skills with herbs, and we call ourselves herbalists.

This skill is an inheritance and is also highly developed amongst the wandering people of the world, especially the Gypsies, Bedouin Arabs and the American and Mexican Indians (nomadic people known to me, and there are many others in lands to which so far I have not travelled). I have sought herbal knowledge from those wandering tribes, living with them and loving them, and much that I have learnt can be found in this book and in my earlier herbal for farm and stable animals.

This twentieth century has seen a universal revival of and interest in herbal medicine. For herbal remedies were fast fading from memory; thirty years ago, when I began writing about herbs for veterinary use, I was quite alone; now thousands are at my side. Further, herbs are to an increasing extent coming back into human orthodox medicine. Many have always held their place there.

Mankind cannot forsake herbs. They are promised in the Bible to the human race, and that promise is well known, for it is proudly quoted in almost every herbal. In the Old and New Testaments there are over a dozen mentions of herbs or medicinal trees of value to mankind, for food or medicine. That our forefathers valued a herb garden is shown in Ahab's plea to Naboth (1 Kings xxi, 2): 'Give me thy vineyard that I may have it for a garden of herbs, because it is near unto my house.'

Man can never excel Nature in medicine manufacture, for she makes the best ones. There is a herb or several herbs to cure or relieve every ailment of man and animal, bird and insect; and herbs applied in agricultural practice will even cure crops of their diseases.

The human race should make a study of herbs and not be content to remain ignorant of a medicine which is man's rightful inheritance, and which has only become lost to men through their ignorance and laziness and their departure from natural living. People should not be content to pay high prices for chemical medicines, which are seldom beneficial to the human body because they are unnatural, and which are very often harmful, their total effects being unknown: instead they should learn to know the wild medicinal plants — the herbs — which are free for the gathering. Teeming in the countryside, the world over, are medicinal herbs and edible plants; it shows disbelief in the power of God to pass them by.

My two children are now grown up and have never had other than herbal treatments in their lives, and have always taken an abundance of wild herbs and fruits in their daily diet. They are both Nature children, enjoying rugged health. When my son was a child, in Spain, his leg was cut almost to the bone by falling jagged blocks from a newly built wall. I healed this injury speedily, using only rosemary. Rosemary has remained my favourite herb ever since, and I use it more than any other herb and cultivate it wherever I live. It was also a favourite of a queen of Hungary, and a lotion from it was known to the gypsies as 'The Queen of Hungary's

Water'. It was sold by Hungarian gypsies on their far travels, and won worldwide fame for its healing properties.

In Israel, where I have lived for many years, I have learnt to make much use of rue. Its medicinal properties have proved so excellent in my herbal work, that I can understand why Mahomet chose this herb for his blessing, and why Arabs everywhere plant it in their gardens to protect their homes against 'the Evil Eye'.

My present work is largely in agriculture, and the use of herbs has given me crops and trees of exceptional health and size, which have attracted the interest of the experts, and brought me encouragement from those who believe in natural agriculture. Also by growing bee herbs I have kept my hives of bees entirely disease-free in a region where that lethal bee disease 'Foul brood' has been rife and very close to my hives. My publishers have asked me to write this herbal for general human use, following my several herbals for veterinary medicine, and have left me entirely free to decide as to the kind of herbal to be written.

I have chosen to write a simple book for Everyman, and have tried to select herbs which are quite well known and easy to find or obtain. The poisonous herbs (which also have their uses) I have not included in this book, as in most cases there are similar non-poisonous herbs which can be employed in their stead.

The same applies to the recipes. I have only included simple ones with ingredients easy to obtain. All the herbal treatments in this book are safe and well proved.

For those readers interested in a more detailed study of herbs and herbal treatments, and in the use of trees in medicine, I have my veterinary herbal for farm and stable, with over seventy pages of Materia Medica. All those veterinary treatments can be applied for human use, and have been so applied through many years. This herbal — *Herbal Handbook for Farm and Stable* — is published by Faber and Faber. It is in most libraries for those who want to see what it is about. I was happy and surprised to obtain a good review of that book in such orthodox farming and field publications as *The Farmer's Weekly* and *The Field* (of England).

In this present book are included many new medicinal herbs and herbal treatments of my own discovery, and hitherto unpublished ones that I have collected on my travels. I hope that it may help newcomers to herbs to discover the wonder of herbal medicine. And I hope that for those who already possess herbal knowledge it may provide a little that is new, and help to strengthen their faith and pride in this great and ancient form of healing.

2

Gathering, Preparing and Preserving Herbs

The most healthful way to use herbs is to gather them fresh from the countryside, or fresh from the herb garden. However, as the majority of herbs are not ever-green some drying and storing is necessary to keep supplies available for medicines throughout the year, especially in hot, dry, climates, where the green period of plant-life is brief.

For gathering of herbs the following rules should be followed.

A general law is that all plants should be gathered during the time when they are at the peak of their growth, usually during the spring and early summer months. The best gathering hours are in the early morning after evaporation of dew. Herbs gathered when dew-wet are not suitable for drying, as they will turn mouldy. The same applies to rain-wet herbs. Also, when gathering for drying it is best to take the herbs at the time of the month when the moon is waning, in the early days of the waning. At such time there is less sap in the foliage and stems, and the herbs dry more speedily.

The following rules are applicable to the different parts of plants required for medicinal use:

LEAVES. Leaves should be picked when young. Newly opened leaf buds possess concentrated medicinal powers. Yellowed, faded, leaves, mottled or insect-bitten ones, should not be used. Snip off all stalks.

17

FLOWERS. Flowers should be gathered in their first opening and before being much visited by bees and other insects. Faded, wilting and insect-eaten flowers should not be picked. As with leaves, snip off stalks when required for drying.

SEEDS. Seeds should be left to sun-ripen as much as possible, ripening on the plant, but watch should be kept to ensure gathering before seed dispersal by wind or other means. Yellowing leaves are often an indication of ripened seeds.

ROOTS. The best time to gather roots for drying is when the sap rises in the early spring, although they may also be taken after the plant sheds its leaves in the autumn or winter. Gather when the moon is waxing full, the roots are then more tender.

BARKS. Barks, as with roots, should be gathered in the early spring or autumn. So as not to damage the shrubs or trees, bark should be taken from the big branches only, which can be sawn off the shrub or tree before the outer bark (and sometimes the inner layers) are collected from them.

Note. It is necessary to *give a warning* nowadays, concerning chemical poison sprays, used on weeds and other herbs. When gathering herbs, care should be taken that they have not been sprayed. Now that poison spraying is often operated from the air, the danger to medicinal herbs is considerable.

PRESERVATION OF HERBS

There are a few simple rules to follow in order to preserve herbs so that they will keep in good condition from season to season. Herbs well preserved can be used up to two years after collecting, when they should be replaced by fresh supplies. Do not merely throw out the old herbs as rubbish; sprinkle them around the most valued garden plants as a tonic, for they will do much further good when used in that way (see Chapter 5).

The main rule in preserving herbs is only to use good-quality material. Therefore all blighted, faded, insect-eaten herbs should be avoided when gathering. The next rule is to make sure of pre-dryness. Herbs to be preserved should not be damp from rain, dew, frost or snow. Also garden herbs being gathered for pressing should not have been watered since the previous day.

LEAVES AND FLOWERS. Herbs dry well in thin brown-paper bags, necks left open, pegged on rope lines. That way can have contact with moderate sunlight. Or can be hung in medium-size bunches, about four large handfuls of herb to a bunch. The bunches are suspended in a cool dry shed or beneath trees, where there is a good flow of air, or spread on tables or shelves and turned frequently. Drying flat between sheets of soft white paper (such as 'shelf' paper), but without pressing, is another method. Herbs can also be dried by layering on fine-mesh wire netting or on closely laid canes, placed on floor or dry ground, and covered with cotton gauze held in place with dust-free stones.

In cold climates, the weak sunlight of early morning and late afternoon can be used directly on the herbs to speed their drying. Hot sunlight causes fading and loss of medicinal properties, and therefore herbs should be protected against this when cut for drying off the plant. When herbs are sun-dried on the plant itself their medicinal properties are diminished but not greatly harmed: this is the easiest way.

Many peasants and gypsies leave herbs to dry on the plant, and cut their herbs direct from the rooted thing, wind- and sun-dried. Sap of shrubs and cacti, and plant resins and juices, especially that of the opium poppy, are taken direct from the herb, to be used fresh, and then made into concoctions such as opium cake.

In cold climates, heat from fire may be necessary to dry plants fully. Only very slow, gentle heat should be used, for quick drying is destructive to the health of all herbs. Just as seeds must be left to ripen naturally and slowly if they are to retain life and be able to germinate when sown, so likewise the life forces of herbs must not be damaged by strong heat.

SEEDS OR FRUITS. Treat as leaves and flowers. When possible dry without removing from the plant, taking care not to lose the seeds by over-early wind dispersal.

The larger fruits can be sun-dried as advised for leaves and flowers in cool climates — or in sunless climates they can be sliced, stones are removed, and remainder is dried off slowly in an oven, using only gentle heat and keeping the door slightly open. Fruits should be turned frequently. When fully dried they should be stored under airtight conditions. Strong canvas bags are best, with the necks tightly tied, and placed in a damp-free area. Dried lavender layered between dried fruits is a preservative.

ROOTS AND BARKS. All dirt and dust must be removed before careful drying; some artificial heat will be necessary in cold climates. Turn frequently during drying.

STORAGE. Herbs can be successfully dried, but then spoilt by careless storage. When herbs are fully dry they can be stored in brown-paper bags, the necks tied with raffia. Or the herbs can be broken into pieces and stored in jars or tins.

The finest containers for medicinal herbs are those old-fashioned tall jars of darkened glass with tight-fitting glass stoppers, as used in chemists' shops. For such storage the herbs are broken small and not packed too tightly.

As I think I have told readers, I am a traveller and cannot take heavy jars along with me. I use strong brown-paper bags tightly tied and find such storage satisfactory. For extra protection I put the paper bags in strong cotton sugar sacks, washed free of all sugar. When the cotton sacks are tightly packed with the paper bags of herbs, the necks are then well tied with fine twisted wire. The sacks then have to be hung from wires arranged in such a way that rodents cannot climb down or drop down on to them. For rodents know well the value of medicinal herbs, seeds, roots, etc. and will eat them and spoil them by contamination.

Care should be taken against spoiling by insects such as beetles, moths, ants and mites of various kinds, which also seek out stored medicinal herbs, since some of the beneficial properties are available to them. In fact, storage is the most difficult part of preserving medicinal herbs, and care must be given to the herbs at all times. In hot climates vermin are especially troublesome. In cold climates there is the danger of mildew.

Quick-freezing method

To quick-freeze herbs, first blanch in boiling water for one minute, then plunge immediately into iced water. Drain through a colander, and then seal quickly in aluminium foil, and put in freezer in refrigerator; keep there until required. This method is good for preserving culinary herbs for flavouring food. It destroys the medicinal powers, and therefore is limited in its use. Also, aluminium does not improve the health of herbs, nor of foods kept within it.

Neither plastic nor nylon should be used for storage of fresh herbs, nor for longtime storage of dried herbs. These are not healthful and spoil the vitality of herbs.

Preparation of herbs

GENERAL. The making of medicines from herbs is a simple process, especially when it is the leaves, flowers or seeds which are used. Of course many of the medicinal leaves, flowers and seeds can be eaten raw by man, and that is the best way to utilize them. But since many medical herbs are unpleasant in taste and extremely bitter, it is usual to take them in the form of a medicinal 'tea' or brew. Dried herbs have twice the strength of fresh, therefore when using fresh, larger amounts should be taken.

Brews, Standard Brew

Leaves and flowers should be snipped off the stalks, and big leaves should be cut into smaller pieces with scissors. This cutting always helps release of juices.

The herbs, freshly gathered or dried, should be placed in an enamel, steel or earthenware pan and the required amount of cold water added. Then there should be heating over a gentle flame until boiling point is almost reached. Keep on the heat for approximately three minutes but do not boil, then remove from the heat and allow the herb to steep (brew) for at least three hours before use. Overnight steeping is best.

Do not strain the herbs; leave them in the pan, or pour the unstrained liquid into a glass jar or a pot. For the longer the herb brews, the better it becomes.

Straining is not necessary, as the herbs settle to the bottom of the vessel and the clear liquid can then be drawn off as required.

Throughout the heating time keep the pot covered in order to prevent escape of vital properties in the steam. Also keep covered during the steeping period and throughout use. The pan lid can be used, slightly raised to admit a little air (otherwise speedy fermentation will ensue). When the brew is stored in jars or pots, a cotton cloth should be tied over the herbal liquid, to admit air but exclude dust and vermin.

Keeping time for brewed herbs is usually three days, less in hot climates. In hot climates always put the herbal liquids to stand out-of-doors in the cooler night air to reduce fermentation. Fermentation does not matter when the herb is required for external use. Fine bubbles seen in the brew after it has stood cold for several days indicate fermentation.

STANDARD BREW. There will be frequent references to this, in the next chapter particularly. General quantities are one large (man-size) handful of dried herbs to two cups of water, prepared as instructed above. This is known as the *Standard Brew*. For more exact measurements of some individual herbs, the following chapter, 'Materia Medica', should be studied.

Seeds, Roots and Barks

SEEDS. When seeds are not eaten raw, they can be placed on flannel, watered, and put in a warm place until germination, which is indicated by cracking of the skin and sprouting white points of root and shoot occurs; they are then ready for use. Or some seeds can be made into a brew, as already described.

Some seeds can be lightly roasted and finely ground, to make them more palatable.

ROOTS. Careful washing to remove all dirt is the first essential. Some roots can be eaten raw, after fine grating. Others, also after some cutting, should be prepared as with leaves and flowers, only in the case of roots there should be some boiling, until quite soft; this can take from a quarter of an hour to one hour, dependent on the plant from which the roots are taken. As with leaves and flowers, keep covered throughout, and then allow to brew in a similar way. Roots usually (except the Solanaceae family) resist fermentation longer than leaves and flowers and therefore can be kept longer when brewed.

BARKS. A few may be eaten raw, but in general they require to be made into a brew, using boiling heat as for roots. When the inner bark layers are required for use, they call for individual preparation, as will be described in Chapter 3.

Cold herbal brews

As I have already said, many leaves, fruits, seeds and some roots, of herbs, can be eaten raw by man. I have evolved a simple method of using many of the unpalatable ones without cooking, for I believe in keeping as close as possible to nature. The wild animals and birds and insects make much use of medicinal herbs, and they do not use fire to prepare them. It is possible for man also to use bitter herbs without heating in water. Milk is the medium used. Raw milk has great powers of absorption, and is itself, when from herbivorous animals, merely vegetable matter in suspension.

Nothing more is necessary than to chop the herbs finely and place them in cold milk and let them stand for four or more hours. Use one heaped tablespoon of herbs to every cup of milk. Keep covered with a muslin or other porous cloth. Pound and press the herbs into the milk before use, then strain and drink. Unpasteurized milk is best. Remove top cream then add herbs.

Some herbs, especially the aromatic ones such as sage, basil, thyme, chervil, etc. also gorse blossoms and rose petals, can be sun-infused, that is to say, left for two days exposed to hot sunlight, shining down into shallow dishes of water; glass dishes are best.

Tincture of herbs

Many herbs can be made into tinctures with the addition of alcohol, cheap surgical spirit or vinegar.

A general mixture is 2 ounces of the powdered herb to one quart of the spirit or liquid used. Make in a glass jar or jars with tight-fitting lids as used for bottling fruit. Lids must be fully airtight. When possible prepare in full sunlight otherwise choose warm place. Shake the bottle many times daily. Making herbal tincture takes about two weeks. When ready, store in a dark place.

Essence of herbs

Essences are made by dissolving 1 to 2 ounces of the essential oil extracted from the herb, in 1 quart of alcohol, surgical spirit or vinegar. Store in a dark place. Essences are for external use. Flower and leaves essences can also be made by filling half a glass bottle with finely crushed herbs and topping up with cheap quality cologne. To every half pint cologne, add 2 teaspoons vinegar, 1 teaspoon castor oil. Infuse in a warm place, shake well night and morning.

Essential oils of herbs

The well-known oils such as oil of eucalyptus, camphor, lavender, can be obtained from most pharmacies. The more unusual oils such as rosemary, thyme, rue, wormwood, etc. have to be obtained by mail from special herbal firms. At the time of writing I do not know of any suppliers in Europe other than a few wholesale druggists who only supply large quantities for commerce, not small amounts for personal use. For years now I have made my own oils, and these have proved quite satisfactory.

Aromatic herbs such as those listed above, from rosemary to wormwood — and I also make oil of lavender and roses and balm — are finely crushed. A common mincing machine can be used, but I prefer the old traditional way of pounding the herbs to a fine pulp, using two stones, one hollow, the other pointed. I place the herbs in a hollow stone and pound them with the pointed stone. A coffee-pounder can be used, but that is usually of metal, and I prefer stone, which should not be too porous.

Two tablespoons of the pounded herb are then placed into a

half-pint bottle, and the bottle is filled three-quarters full with a fine oil, such as corn- or sunflower-oil and a tablespoonful of pure vinegar. The bottle is corked and placed in hot sunlight. The contents are shaken daily. At midday I change the position of the bottles so that they are always in the sunlight. After approximately three weeks, the oils are ready for use. To make strong oil, the clear oil should be strained off every five days, for three weeks; the herbal residue is then shaken from the bottle and all oil pressed from it, then newly pounded herbs should be added to the strained oil.

In lands where there is no strong sunlight, artificial heat must be used. The tightly corked bottles, which must not be more than three-quarters full, are placed in a double pan of water, and heated gently for several hours, always keeping the water below boiling point. The heating must be repeated daily for a week or so, until the required strength of oil is obtained, i.e the oil should be strong enough to hold perceptibly the scent of the plant used when applied, as a test, on the skin of your arm.

Herbal Poultices

Poultices are one of the most important ways of applying herbs to the human body. They have been used since ancient times and are still an unsurpassed method of drawing out toxins from the skin and other organs of the body, for reducing inflammation, for curing sores, and for dissolving small cysts and tumours.

Linseed poultice. This is one of the best known, and it deserves its popularity. In the class of 'common' poultice, it is for general use. A linseed poultice is made as follows. Warm a basin by rinsing it out gently with water just off the boil. Then pour into the warmed bowl a pint of boiling water. Using the left hand, sprinkle into the boiling water a quarter pound of linseed. Meanwhile, with a strong wooden spoon stir the mixture well until a smooth dough is produced, stirring quickly to prevent lumpiness. When the dough is made, stir into it a half-ounce of olive oil (for treatment of tumours use castor

25

oil). Then spread thickly on a piece of warmed linen, using speed so as to retain the heat of the mixture. Then the ends are folded over and the poultice applied where needed. Or the linseed meal can be used hot, pressed into tightly-sewn cotton bags. For a 'drawing' poultice, raw, grated, or boiled mashed carrots, or turnips, can be added to the linseed mixture. Do not press either the carrots or turnips; retain all their juice, and mix speedily into the linseed to give a thin mash, which is then applied directly where needed, or used within cotton bags.

Precautions should always be taken against the poultices being applied too hot.

Charcoal poultice. A 'cleansing' poultice; raw grated, or boiled mashed carrots or turnips, made into a paste with vegetable charcoal, the charcoal to be in fine powder form. Use enough carrots or turnips to form a paste, and apply direct to the skin where required.

Garlic or Onion poultice. Grate finely, or boil, a quarter pound of garlic or a half pound of onions, and add to this the crumb of a pound wheaten loaf, soaked in whey or cold milk. Apply direct to the body area.

Poppy-heads poultice. A 'soothing' poultice. Boil a handful of fresh or dried poppy heads (any species of poppy), in water, strain, and add the above described linseed meal to this to stiffen it, and spread direct on the skin where required. As well as soothing, this natural-opium poultice draws out toxic matter from infected wounds.

Herbal Poultice Bandages. Made by sprinkling powdered slippery elm bark (obtained from herbalists) into a small bowlful of boiling brew until a thin paste is made. The brew is made from the chosen herb for the illness under treatment. The herb, finely cut, should be left in the water and worked into the paste. This is all then spread, warm, on to a linen bandage, for applying directly on to the wound, gathering, or whatever is being treated. Or a green pulp of the chosen herbs, in their raw state, can be worked into slightly liquefied slippery elm powder, pounding all into a smooth paste to be applied cold to the linen bandage, and then used as described above.

The herbs adder's-tongue, chickweed, gypsy-wort, St. John's wort, violet and wood betony are especially good for making the herbal poultice bandages.

A Standard Herbal Fomentation. Mix together two handfuls each of fresh wormwood, rue, chamomile, and half a handful of bay leaves — rather less of dried herbs. Boil well in a quart of water. Allow to steep overnight. Apply hot by dipping flannel into the re-heated solution and bind firmly over the area to be treated. It is a proved remedy for painful and hard abscesses, boils, gatherings, sores, and aching areas of the body.

Herbal Pills

One can easily make raw herbal pills for immediate use. Pound fresh herbs into a pulp, binding them into a firm paste with molasses or thick honey and fine cornflour. Roll into small balls and place each inside a piece of clean white tissue paper or thin piece of cotton wool, lightly damped with cold water. The outer covering is swallowed along with the contents — paper is only wood pulp, a favourite diet of goats! Cotton wool is also plant matter, from the flower of the cotton plant.

Prepared Herbs

Those who have no land on which to grow herbs, and are far from countryside where herbs can be gathered wild, can obtain them in dried form from health shops, which are now to be found in many towns. Not all the herbs I discuss will be available, but shops will often supply an alternative. In England, most health food shops now stock a range of herbs, also Culpeper shops; in the U.S.A. there are the Indiana Botanic Gardens, Ind., and Walnut Acres, Penns Creek, Pa. The Wild Flower Remedies of the late Dr. Bach are very suitable for children; they treat the human soul as well as the body. His books are published by The C. W. Daniel Company, Ltd., 1 Church Path, Saffron Walden, Essex, CB10 1JP, U.K.

I do not supply plain herbs, but like most herbalists, I have a few preparations made to my own formula, for veterinary use.

27

Preparations may be obtained from Larkhall Natural Health Ltd, Forest Road, Charlbury, Oxon OX7 3HH, UK. (Not licensed for USA.)

3

Herbal Materia Medica

This chapter gives medicinal and culinary herbs in alphabetical order. Over two hundred herbs are included, with their uses and dosage. Many of the herbs are not to be found in any known Herbal, and several are of the author's own discovery. Habitat is briefly described, and a description of the herb is given, with its use to man, and the dosage in which it should be taken.

With every herb is given the official Latin name as well as its common one. As the Latin names are international, a book on wild flowers in any language, *with illustrations*, will enable readers to identify the herbs if they are not already known to them.

Although this book will be published in Great Britain, I have not confined myself to European herbs: they are taken from the countries which I have visited in many parts of the world. However, most of them, with the exception of the cacti perhaps, can be obtained almost everywhere.

All the herbs given are safe and well proved.

The standard description of 'herb' is: 'a seed plant which does not develop woody persistent tissue (as that of a tree), but is more or less soft or succulent and is used either for medicinal purposes or for its scent or flavour.'

This is a very broad description, for herbs can be food also. The cereals, for instance, are herbs in more than mere 'flavour'; they nourish those who partake of them, and most of them also possess many healing properties. Nevertheless, it will be seen that there is some degree of emphasis on perennial flowering plants.

However, in order to keep this book within reasonable proportions for household use, which is my purpose for this herbal, I have excluded trees, with the exception of a few which are more shrubs than trees, and are so valuable to mankind as healers of their common ills that I was unwilling to leave them out, though they cannot properly be defined as 'herbs'. At some future date I hope to write a short book on medicinal trees, for their healing powers are many and wonderful. I have included many trees in my earlier herbal for veterinary use.

The herbs in this book can be used in the way the reader chooses: taken raw, infused in milk by the 'cold' method, made into a Standard brew (see page 22) in heated water, or made into pills — all fully described elsewhere.

I have used primitive dosage for the herbs in this chapter, 'handfuls, cupfuls, spoonfuls' and so on: Only in my chapter of Recipes, Chapter 4, have I given mostly scale weight measures, for in the recipes one needs to be more exact: whereas with the crude herbs precise amounts either in the making or in the taking as medicine are not essential. With chemical medicines over-dosage may be dangerous, whereas with herbs a little above or below the general dose does not matter at all. Herbalists do not travel around with weighing-scales. The primitive measures of hands and cups and spoons are general, and everyone will use his own judgement.

The dosage for infants can be adjusted from the adult dose. Infants require a little less than half the adult dose, but again, the exact quantities are not of importance.

ADDER'S TONGUE (*Ophioglossum vulgatum*. Filices). Found in uncultivated fields and waste places. A fern plant, but possessing dark, smooth, oval leaves, and a distinctive flowering part forming a thin, hard spike, which resembles the tongue of the adder. It is grouped with Moonwort in some classifications, and some exclude it from the ferns.

Use. A famed wound herb, for external use. A handful of the leaf and spike are heated gently in olive oil, two average-size cupfuls of oil to one handful of herb. Heated below boiling point for half an hour. Or the raw herb can be pounded into common toilet cold cream, one tablespoon of herb to four ounces of cold cream.

Apply to all wounds, sores, bruises, ulcers and chilblains. The best way of applying is to spread the Adder's Tongue ointment thickly on clean adder's tongue leaves, and bind into place, using cotton bandages.

AGRIMONY (*Agrimonia eupatoria.* Rosaceae). Found in hedgerows, uncultivated fields and heathland. Thornless leaves of rose-form, and also rose-form flowers, yellow, growing in spikes, and having a distinctive apricot scent.

Use. Its chief use is as a remedy for jaundice, from which the plant takes its Latin name. It is also a cough and asthma remedy. Being astringent it is useful in dropsy.

Dose. A handful of the herb brewed in one and a half pints of water or buttermilk. Reduce by slow heating to one pint. Or taken raw in pill form. Two dessertspoons of the pulped raw herb made into pills, and taken morning and night, about six pills per dose. A weak brew is a remedy for earache and will dissolve hard wax when dropped warm into the ears.

ALDER (*Alnus glutinosa.* Betulaceae). Alders indicate the presence of water. Grows as a small tree in damp places, mainly in marshes and along river-sides. It has a thick trunk, grows shrub height, and bears shiny oval leaves and flowers of green catkin form. (Male ones pendulous, female erect.)

Use. Both leaves and bark are used. Being astringent, cooling and soothing, the shrub is much employed to reduce swellings, alleviate dropsy, and was an old aid in gangrene. It makes a good poultice, and is effective to relieve swollen and inflamed breasts.

The Red Indians have long used alder leaves inside their

moccasins, to keep their feet cool and enable them to travel long distances. Country people use fresh alder leaves inside their boots to soothe aching and burning feet.

For use as a poultice, merely pulp up a handful of leaves, moisten with warm milk, and bind over the place needing treatment.

Dose. One teaspoonful of the powdered bark brewed in one cupful of water by 'Standard' method, or make into pills; one or two dessertspoons of the leaves, taken morning and night, as a remedy against diarrhoea, dropsy and general weakness.

ALFALFA (*Medicago sativa*. Leguminosae). Usually called Lucerne. Found in pasture-land, wild and cultivated. It is a perennial plant, with small grey-green leaves, and small purple, pea-shaped flowers, sometimes whitish. This is a very popular fodder herb, and it is equally good for human use.

Use. Rich in vitamins and minerals it is a fine tonic, kidney cleanser and alkalizer of the whole system. Known for the speed that it gives to race-horses, it is likewise effective for all athletes.

Dose. Take as a salad herb, cut small. A small handful twice daily. Or make into tea, the fresh herb or dried. A popular American drink, it is flavoured with orange peel, lemon peel, mint and honey and drunk very cold.

ALOES (*Aloe communis*, or *socotrina*. Liliaceae). South Africa, Barbados, Socotra. This is a plant of dry, sandy and rocky regions, and is also much cultivated in gardens. The leaves grow in wands and are tall, fleshy and spike-toothed to protect them from grazing animals. The Indians call the aloes 'wands of heaven' because of the wonderful medicinal powers. Legend says that it is the only plant which came direct from the Garden of Eden.

It is the solid juice which is most used in medicine. The juice is pressed from the leaves, sun-dried and exported all over the world as a powerful laxative and blood-cleanser.

Use. Treatment of constipation, intestinal worms, indigestion, lack of appetite.

Dose. Two to four grains of powdered juice, i.e. about one small or large pinch, taken in a half cupful of warm milk sweetened with molasses or honey.

Externally: to cure wounds, sores, ulcers in the mouth and to allay heat rash or poison ivy rash, apply the fresh, cool, gummy juice direct from the fresh leaves, first shaving off the spiked borders and then cutting the leaves crosswise to release the juice. A famed mastitis cure.

ANGELICA (*Archangelica officinalis*. Umbelliferae). Found in damp and woodland places and cultivated in gardens. It is a rather hairy plant with ferny leaves and umbels of white flowers of most powerful and fragrant scent.

Use. The leaves, broad leaf-stalks and roots are used, especially stalks. Also the seeds. For all digestive troubles, including colic and heartburn, it is a good cordial made into a drink with honey (Standard brew). Candied angelica stalks are a popular sweetmeat in France and Spain, and the candy is valued for its tonic properties and for fertility.

Dose. The seeds are used as a mild tea, one teaspoonful of seed to one and a half cups of water to bring up wind in infants and to soothe disordered stomachs. The roots, more powerful, can be used. Also the tea is a good eye tonic, strain it carefully before use. It is important not to confuse this plant with Hemlock, of the same family, which has a poisonous principle, conine.

ANISE (*Pimpinella anise*. Umbelliferae). Found in hedgerows and fields and on rocky hillsides. Distinguished by its feathery leaves of brilliant green, and umbels of creamy flowers forming yellow seeds. The whole plant is highly aromatic and pleasant smelling. The anise of gardens flowers in July and in a good season, seeds are ripe in late August. The 'star anise' (*Illicium verum*) a tropical, Asiatic plant related to the magnolia, supplies many of the seeds in commerce. *Pimpinella* is the true aniseed. The seeds and extracted oil of the plant are used as flavouring and medicine, and can be purchased from most chemists and some grocers.

Use. Similar to angelica. Only it is more powerfully tonic than angelica, and is used as a tonic to flavour cakes and rye bread.

33

Dose. In digestive ailments chew one teaspoon of the seed before meals, three times daily. For babies, make a mild tea, using one teaspoon of seed to one cup of water, and give several teaspoons of the tea before meals, or if bottle fed, then add to the milk.

For bread and cakes, a heaped teaspoon of anise seed to every pound of flour.

ASPARAGUS (*Asparagus officinalis*. Liliaceae). Found on banksides and in woodlands, its fleshy, scaly, sweet-tasting shoots are well known. From the shoots develop the delicate but quite spiky asparagus fern. It is cultivated in gardens for its good-tasting shoots. In the Middle East it can be gathered wild in considerable quantities, after the first rains .

In Galilee I have a contest with the wild animals to gather the healthful, delicious shoots of wild asparagus before all are eaten up. The shoots contain a unique crystalline principle called asparagin.

Use. There is no known herb which acts more powerfully on the urinary system, nor any herbs more beneficial for this purpose. It is a proved remedy for all derangements and obstructions of the kidneys and bladder. It also acts favourably upon the lymphatic system. A remedy for dropsy, jaundice, gall troubles. It is also aperient.

Dose. A handful of the shoots eaten before meals. For medicinal purposes eat the shoots raw. When not available, the canned shoots also possess some medicinal properties. Or a tea can be made from the fern (see 'Standard brew'). Take a cupful, sweetened with honey, morning and night.

BALM (*Melissa officinalis*. Labiatae). Found in woodlands, it has rather rough foliage of a dark shade, and very fragrant. Its flowers are hooded and small, white shading to yellow. Beloved by bees from which its name *melissa* is derived. This was the favoured herb of the great medieval herbalist Paracelsus, who sold the remedy to kings as an elixir of life. The plant is said to safeguard against early senility and impotency. It possesses tannin and a pungent oil, from which the Arabs, who love this plant, make a perfume. It is a well-known

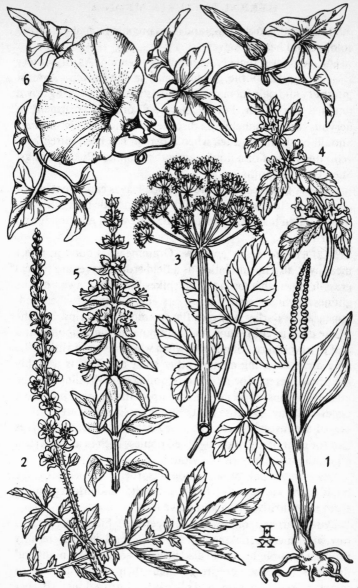

Plate I. 1. Adder's Tongue 2. Agrimony 3. Angelica
4. Balm   5. Basil   6. Bindweed

monastery herb and monks and nuns prepare from it a fragrant cologne and healing salves.

Use. As a fever remedy, to promote sweating. As a dysentery remedy and to soothe griping pains in the bowels. Against infertility and painful or delayed menstruation. To bring down retained after-birth. For all uterine disorders. Treatment of nervous disorders including disordered mind and nightmares. Should be drunk as a tea when a person has been bitten by a venomous insect or a dog or any other animal. Place amongst linen to deter moths.

Dose. A tablespoon of the chopped leaves can be eaten raw twice daily. It is a palatable herb and I include it in our daily salads and in teas. Also, infused in white wine, add honey and raisins.

BARLEY (*Hordeum pratense.* Gramineae). Found in moist meadows, also in cultivation as a field crop. Leaves are typical grass-form, rather broad. The spikes have long awns on the glumes, which give barley its characteristic 'bearded' appearance. Barley is of pale flaxen colour when ripe, and the whole crop in cultivation has a shimmering light upon it and makes a typical rustling sound when wind-blown, owing to the long awns brushing against other spikelets. This is a highly medicinal cereal, being blood-cooling and healing to the internal organs, especially acting upon the kidneys in a most beneficial way. Because of its blood-cooling property, this is one of the favoured cereals of the Arabs, both for themselves and for their prized thoroughbred ponies. Rich in all minerals, especially iron; very rich in vitamin B.

Use. Treatment of all blood disorders, ailments of the bladder and kidneys, as a food for invalids and infants, and as a general nutritive food and nerve tonic.

Dose. Barley is one of the few cereals which can be eaten raw, after merely soaking in water for several days, preferably exposed to sunlight. It can also be eaten soaked overnight and then lightly boiled, or fire-parched, then ground and eaten merely mixed with water and olive oil to form a dough (Berber Arab method), or ground into a fine flour and made into bread. The water from boiled and well-squeezed barley, with honey and lemon juice added, makes an excellent drink. A Turkish peasant method of which I make much use for my family and for my hounds, is to soak raw barley grains in water with lumps of the salty sheep or goat milk cheese. The whey and salt from the cheese soften the grain and also make it very palatable. Soak for two days when it is then ready for eating, without any cooking. Keep covered with a fine mesh cloth.

BASIL (*Ocimum basilicum*. Labiatae). Found in woodland and on banksides. Shiny oval leaves and whorls of small white hooded flowers. Known as 'Sweet Basil' the plant has an alluring scent, and was once much used in White Magic. I can believe it. This herb fascinates me and I make much use of it as food and medicine. I use the whorls of flowers, steeped in olive oil, to flavour olives. The Jews hold sprays of basil in their hands to give them strength during religious fasts. It is *L'herbe Royale* of France, and was fed to the young princes as a regular item of diet.

Use. It is a powerful tonic, stimulant and nerve remedy. Will relieve nausea and severe vomiting. A remedy for indigestion. Externally applied as a rub, is used against the bites of snakes, scorpions and poisonous spiders. Is an insecticide.

BILBERRY (*Vaccinium myrtillus*. Vacciniaceae). Found on heaths and dry hillsides. Leaves small, shaded from green to red-brown, fleshy pinkish flowers forming round and very juicy, pungent-tasting dark blue berries, very cool to the mouth and throat. The plant is highly astringent. It yields a useful blue dye from the berries. The gypsies make a tonic tea from the young leaves.

Use. To check prolonged dysentery and vomiting. A good drink in fevers. A mild worm remedy. Treatment of all nervous ailments. Externally as a gargle or wash for throat and sinus ailments. For treatment of piles.

Dose. A handful or more of the berries three times daily, or a small cupful of the pressed juice morning and night. For a tea, take one tablespoon of the leaves to one and a half cupfuls of water. For external use, crush the berries and apply or make a strong brew from the leaves, two tablespoons to two cupfuls of water. Remember when using the berries externally that their juice stains clothing.

BINDWEED (*Convolvulus arvensis*. Convolvulaceae). Found in hedgerows and pastures as a climbing plant. Has heart-shaped leaves and thin, twisting stems. Flowers are white, pale pink or blue, and are bell-shaped.

Use. As a tonic and cleanser of the blood. Also helpful in dropsy. A fertility herb.

Dose. Three or four flowers eaten in salad twice daily. Or a brew from the twisting stems. Of the brew, take a tablespoon morning and night.

BISTORT (*Polygonum bistorta*. Polygonaceae). This plant of the buckwheat family is found in moist meadows. It is distinguished by its flesh-coloured flowers on short stalks with bracts at base, many jointed stems and large twisted root. The root is the part used.

Use. The drying bitter root is unrivalled as an astringent herb and is therefore excellent for gargles and as a cure for prolonged dysentery. Used as a wash or gargle for ailments of mouth, throat and ears, popular for treatment of internal ulcers. Will expel worms.

Dose. Pieces of root in all to measure about six inches, finely sliced and made up into a brew using a half-pint of water. Boil for five minutes, keeping covered as always in herbal brews. For internal use, take two tablespoons of the brew before meals.

Externally, merely utilize the lotion as a gargle or wash. The dried, powdered, root makes a good remedy to stem serious bleeding from wounds or for treatment of haemorrhages.

BLACKBERRY (*Rubus fruticosus*. Rosaceae). Found in hedgerows, woodlands and by stream-sides. It is well known, widespread, and is distinguished by its prickly foliage and stems, white, rose-form flowers, and big, juicy, black fruits — the familiar Blackberry. A plant rich in medicinal properties.

38

Use. To cool the blood, nerve tonic, laxative. A cure for anaemia, general debility.

Dose. Eat as many of the raw, ripe berries as desired. For infants make a juice from the berries. A Standard brew of the leaves, a cupful sweetened with honey, is a cure for blood and skin disorders. Also apply the brew as an external lotion for cure of eczema. Other species of Rubus share the same properties, namely raspberry, loganberry, dewberry.

BONESET (*Eupatorium perfoliatum*. Compositae). Found in damp places. Has rough and hairy stems. Leaves also rather hairy. Flowers are white or creamy and very numerous. Named after King Eupator, King of Pontus, who discovered and extolled the medicinal uses of this plant. Its common name of boneset came from the success obtained with this plant in speeding the setting of broken bones and soothing aching ones.

Use. It is useful in all forms of fevers and colds. In all bone weakness from rickets to tender or aching bones.

Dose. A Standard brew of the flowering tops or leaves. A half cupful morning and night.

BORAGE (*Borago officinalis*. Boraginaceae). Found in fields and woods, likes dry ground. Leaves are rough, flowers of wheel-form and brilliant blue shade. It is used by Arabs as a salad herb — the women eat it to increase their milk when nursing babies. It also has powers against the stings or bites of poisonous creatures.

Use. To strengthen the heart and limbs. Mildly laxative, it is good for ailments of the digestive system. A jaundice remedy. Will increase milk flow. Was once said to cleanse all poisons from the blood resulting from bites or stings from such things as snakes, scorpions, rabid dogs. Such ancient claims must of course be seen in their true perspective as indicators of the herb's prophylactic or curative virtues. Externally it makes an excellent eye lotion and ringworm remedy.

Dose. Eat a small handful of the leaves and flowers, divided into several salad meals, or make a Standard brew and drink as a tea morning and night, a small cupful.

Externally apply the Standard brew as an eye lotion. Pulp the leaves and squeeze the juice on to ringworm patches.

BROOM (*Cytisus scoparius*. Leguminosae). Found on heaths, sandy commons and rocky hillsides. Has tiny oval leaves, and pea-form flowers, yellow in colour, sweetly and strongly-scented. Spanish gypsies make a cologne from the flowers. This plant earned fame in Russia for prevention and cure of rabies. (See note under 'Borage'.) It acts on the lymph and is therefore effective in the treatment of dropsy.

Use. To cure worm-infestation, jaundice and dropsy. To expel poisons from bites by venomous insects. To increase flow of urine in kidney and bladder disease.

Dose. Two tablespoons of broom tops brewed in three-quarters pint of water. Take a tablespoon morning and night. In treatment of hydrophobia it was usual to take a tablespoon every hour. For external use make a strong brew of the twigs as a scalp rub against lice.

BURDOCK (*Arctium lappa*. Compositae). Found on waste places and by roadsides. Is much disliked as a pasture weed, since it clings to wool and spoils its quality. ('Good for nothing', the farmer said, as he made a sweep at the burdock's head.) Has large rhubarb-type leaves, and thistle-like pale purple flowers which form barbed fruits — burs, which adhere to clothing and to the bodies of animals. All parts are medicinal, roots, leaves and burs. Burdock is one of the most valued plants in herbal medicine. It rapidly increases the flow of urine.

Use. Remedy for all blood disorders, including the chronic ones, gout, rheumatism, arthritis, sciatica. Externally, for treatment of burns, scalds, skin irritation, boils, carbuncles, skin parasites.

Dose. Brew one ounce of the root in three-quarters of a pint of water, simmer for a quarter of an hour and then steep for three hours. Bruise and slice the root before adding the water. Take a small cupful, sweetened with honey, night and morning. In chronic blood disorders, take a cupful three times daily. For external use, burns, scalds, skin irritations and parasites, apply as a lotion using a stronger brew.

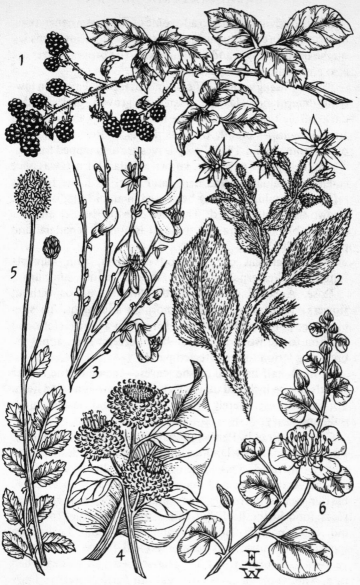

Plate 2. 1. Blackberry   2. Borage   3. Broom
4. Burdock   5. Burnet   6. Caper

It is also advantageous to add some of the burs when making the stronger brew, using more root to the water. For burns lay on the bruised leaves and bind in place. The bruised leaves are also a remedy against ringworm.

BURNET (*Sanguisorba officinalis*. Rosaceae). Found on low-lying damp land. Has tall, branching growth, and crowded dark purple flowers, small. The name of the plant is derived from *sanguis* — blood, from its ability to stem the flow of blood from wounds. The fleshy leaves are also tapped for sap.

Another species of burnet, known as Salad-burnet, was once eaten as a valuable salad herb, and takes its name from its refreshing qualities, having been used in an old English drink known as Cool-Tankard. The properties of burnet are: for healing, blood-cooling and tonic. It is a most beneficial and protective herb.

Use. Treatment of all blood disorders, skin ailments (internal and external treatment), wound healing, sun-burn.

Dose. A Standard brew of the shoots with or without flowers. Take a small cupful morning and night. To stop bleeding: pulp up the herb and spread on a gauze cloth and bind on to the wound. For sun-burn, eczema, etc. apply the brew as a lotion to the affected parts.

Dose. A half-handful of the leaves — some of the flower whorls can be included daily. To be eaten raw as a salad herb. For external use, merely bruise the leaves and flowers into a pulp and apply.

CACTUS (Prickly Pear) (*Opuntia ficus-indica*. Cactaceae). Found on dry rocky land and along borders of deserts, also widely cultivated. This form of cactus is planted as a fence around Arab houses and lands, where it makes an effective barrier against intruders, man and animals, and also provides food in the healthful edible fruits, and fuel from the old, dried portions of the plant and its roots. Leaves are typical cactus form, but very broad and fleshy. Flowers are yellow, rose-form; fruits are pear-shaped and golden when ripe. The whole plant is covered with fine, protective hairs which are highly irritant to the human skin, and must be removed from the fruits by rubbing them in sand and then washing them sand free in running water. All parts of this cactus are medicinal.

Use. Treatment of amoebic dysentery (the flowers are considered a specific remedy). As food and for treatment of wounds and skin ailments (the inner flesh of the leaves). As food and laxative medicine (the fruit).

Dose. The flowers as a treatment for amoebic dysentery are used as follows: a handful of fresh (or less, if dried) flowers to a pint of cold water, bring to the near boil, simmer below boiling point for three minutes, steep for three hours, drink a cupful morning and night. On the third and fourth day of treatment, an enema should be given. The leaves are sliced, stripped of the outer skin, then baked and eaten with lemon, salt and oil. The fruits are freed of the prickles, carefully cut across to remove the outer skin, and eaten raw. The fleshy leaves are also tapped for sap.

CANDYTUFT (*Iberis amara*. Cruciferae). Found on chalky or rocky land, often as an outcast from gardens. Has small-toothed shiny leaves, and tufts of flattish flowers, usually white. Named after Iberia — Spain. Favoured for centuries by the Spanish peasants. The whole plant is medicinal, and formerly it was carefully cultivated for its curative powers in rheumatism and kindred ailments.

Use. Treatment of rheumatism, including the most chronic forms, arthritis, sciatica, gout, Berger's disease, dropsy.

Dose. Make a Standard brew of the whole plant, and take two tablespoons of the brew before meals, or a pinch of the powdered seeds before meals.

CANNABIS (Hemp) (*Cannabis sativa, Cannabis indica*. Moraceae). A wild or cultivated plant. In wild state found on wasteland, alongside pathways and sometimes as a woodland plant. It is a strong-growing weed and is easy to cultivate. Being of a burning and poisonous nature it is mostly resistant to insect pests. Its main use has always been the manufacture of a very strong and unbreakable type of rope, made from the fibre that it produces. It is also misused, with some harmful results, as a narcotic. It possesses palm-shaped, composite leaves, with dark green, shiny, narrow leaflets. The flowers are small, unattractive, feathery, of a yellowish-green colour and grow in spikes. The fruits are male or female and of a bivalvular form. When the stems and leaves are stripped bare this plant has a sinister crocodile look. Indeed, it is one of the world's sinister plants, and has a long association with Lucifer. It is appropriate and significant that the hangman's vile rope is made traditionally from the cannabis plant. People claim many beneficial effects from cannabis (also called marijuana). The medicinal claims are as a cure for various ailments including those of the nervous system. I do accept that externally, because it has burning properties, it can reduce soft tumours, remove warts, soften corns and cure blisters or blistered areas including scalds. But personally my experience of cannabis addicts on my world travels is that it turns normally pleasant humans into objectionable ones, with frayed nerves, unreliable character, bouts of angry (abnormal) behaviour, and with fetid breath because of the severe constipation which this drug causes. Another hazardous effect is to create a craving for sweet foods to try and neutralize the dehydrating and bitter effects of cannabis on the mouth, throat and stomach. This heavy intake of sweet foods sets up a vicious circle, worm infestation can result and the liver may be harmed. That often dangerous condition known as hepatitis is an acknowledged common ailment of heavy consumers of cannabis. Also there is often abnormal, heavy salivation, as unattractive as the ugly, dilated pupils of the eyes of cannabis addicts. The eyes are the mirrors of the soul, and it is significant that this drug spoils the look of the eyes of those who abuse it. In a farmhouse on one of the Spanish Balearic islands, Formentera, I found an old Spanish herbal, dated 1805, and even then there were severe warnings against the harmful effects derived from smoking or eating cannabis. The book stated that this drug creates a craving which often proves very difficult to overcome. Desire for the drug builds up, so that very large doses become necessary to satisfy the taker. The effect of cannabis may at first prove energizing and pleasing to the mind, often giving, like alcohol, escape from reality but prolonged abuse has worse mental effects than alcohol as it makes users very sleepy, disinclined to work, very bad-tempered and often extremely violent. One of the worst results described by cannabis addicts is that they lose their normal sense of time; and while pleasant dreams may be induced by cannabis, terrible dreams are also commonplace and have a disturbing effect. It is very interesting that there is an almost worldwide ban on the use of cannabis as a drug, and I feel that the nations which seek to protect their people's health have very good reason and experience for this ban. I hope that my book will help to support the ban against cannabis, as I've seen many young lives spoilt by this vicious plant.

Use. In rope-making. (The famed rope-soled shoes of Spain, *alpargatas*, are made from cannabis fibre.) As a narcotic drug: the dried leaves, flowers or fruits are chewed or smoked releasing into the blood and nervous system the active principle of the plant, a greenish, oily substance, cannabinol. Externally, to reduce and remove soft growths, including some types of tumours.

Dose. It is strongly recommended not to take any cannabis. Externally: a handful of the leaves pulped and applied fresh. Internally: remember cannabis is a dangerous mind-changer.

CAPER (Thorny caper. *Capparis spinosa*. Capparidaceae). A Mediterranean herb found by waysides and in rocky areas. Greyish shiny foliage and thorny stems. Flowers are beautiful, pale purple with numerous prominent stamens of darker purple. The buds are pickled in vinegar by the Arabs. The fruits are used in the pickle industry. Both buds and fruits are a powerful tonic. Capers stimulate the digestive juices and increase appetite.

Use. A tonic, eaten as a pickle or cooked vegetable. The buds and fruits are used. Capers are good added to mayonnaise. The fruits are sold in bottles in most good groceries. For home-made capers merely gather four handfuls of the young buds, and place in a jar with a pint of natural vinegar and four to five bay leaves, several peeled cloves of garlic. Cap well and shake frequently. When the capers are fully soft (about three weeks) they are ready to eat. The caper vinegar is refreshing and healthful.

CARAWAY (*Carum carvi*. Umbelliferae). Found on dry banks and waste places. It has feathery leaves which emit the well-known anise scent when bruised, umbels of creamy yellow flowers which bear the small, dark, half-moon seeds known in confectionery as well as in medicine. The seed is the part for which the caraway herb is famed, excelling as a tonic for all the organs of digestion. For that reason caraway seed came to be used in cakes and breads. Caraway strengthens and gives tone to the whole digestive tract, and also influences beneficially the liver and gall. The leaves are also edible and medicinal, but much milder than the seeds.

Use. For all the digestive ailments. To expel wind in infants; to expel internal gas and soothe the digestive tract. To increase appetite and sweeten the bowels. To tone the liver and stimulate flow of bile. To take with other laxatives to lessen griping.

Dose. A half-teaspoon of the seeds chewed before meals. For infants a half-teaspoon made into a tea with hot water. Allow to brew and then give the teaspoon of the liquid, warm, before meals. When added to cakes, bread, etc. it has a pleasant aromatic flavour, but cooking greatly diminishes its medicinal properties.

A few sprays of the leaves can be chopped up in salads. The American Indians made a valued embrocation from wild anise or caraway leaves steeped in buffalo oil (a vegetable oil is preferable).

CARROT (*Daucus carota*. Umbelliferae). Found wild in damp places and hedgerows, and cultivated in gardens. There is a poisonous member of the Umbelliferae family much resembling wild carrot, so care should be taken when gathering the wild herb.

The appearance of the garden carrot is well known. The carrot plant possesses great medicinal powers and is one of the herbs recognized by herbalists as being beneficial in cancer treatment.

Use. The garden carrot has a thick, juicy, reddish root; used as food and medicine. As a food it is a tonic and rich in vitamins and minerals. Because of its high tonic properties it has a good effect also on the eyes and is recommended to improve eyesight. A pint to a quart of fresh carrot is much used by herbalists in treatment of cancer. The grated root, made into a fresh poultice and applied to bad wounds, old sores, swellings, tumours, is soothing and curative. Carrot is a remedy for anaemia, jaundice, internal ulcers (the juice), worms (the grated root), styes in eyelids, and twitching eyes (the juice applied), also for kidney and bladder troubles (the grated root eaten or a strong tea made from the leaves). Grated raw carrots eaten daily give relief in painful menstruation. A strong tea of the blossom is effective in dropsy and all lymphatic ailments, also varicose veins. Being rich in a natural insulin, carrots are excellent food and medicine for diabetic patients (though in ignorance, because they are sweet, they are often banned for diabetics).

Dose. There is no specific dose, eat as much *raw* carrot daily as the body will tolerate.

A pint to a quart of the juice is advised in severe illness, such as anaemia, cancer. The leaves are bitter, but a few pieces can be chopped fine and sprinkled on the salad. The flowers should be made into a Standard brew, and a dessertspoonful taken daily before meals. Or a small wineglassful, sweetened with honey, can be taken morning and night.

CASTOR OIL PLANT or CASTOR BEAN (*Ricinus communis*. Euphorbiaceae). Found wild in woodland or pasture, and cultivated in gardens, parks, etc. This shrub sometimes reaches tree proportions. It has palm-like leaves which may span several feet. Its flowers are red and plume-like. The fruit is a bean which yields the well-known pharmacy product, *castor oil*, famed as a speedy purge. Frequent external applications reduce warts and tumours. This small palm was called *Palma Christi* in medieval Latin, when its great healing powers gave it association with one of the most famed of all the healers, Jesus Christ. It is also called 'Christ's Hand', not only because the

47

leaves have resemblance to a human hand outspread, but because the touch of the leaves and the extracted oil from the seeds heal many disorders.

Use. A prompt and powerful laxative. Of great use in poisoning and for removing intestinal worms, including tapeworm. Used externally the leaves make a powerful drawing poultice when bound over wounds, sores, swellings, tumours. The oil is an effective rub for inflamed skin, bruises, to prevent falling hair and to grow new hair (where the hair follicles are not totally withered). Moles are known to desert their burrows when castor oil seeds are sprinkled within.

Dose. Three tablespoons of the oil as a speedy purge for an adult person; less for a child. Castor oil is not recommended for infants. As a poultice, bruise a half dozen leaves, of size big enough to cover the area requiring treatment and bind into place, to exclude air. As a rub, several dessertspoons of the oil. It is best used hot. A good mixture for using as a rub to reduce tumours and to cure skin ailments such as ringworm and mange, is two parts castor oil to one part wine vinegar, used hot, and massaged into the area night and morning. Add a little lemon juice to the spoon before pouring the castor oil into the spoon. It will prevent sticky adherence of the oil to the spoon and subsequent wastage.

CATNIP (*Napeta cataria*. Labiatae). Found in hedges and on waste places. Greyish, strongly scented. Flowers white or pale lavender, hooded. Cats eat the leaves for their medicinal properties and like to roll in this plant — hence its name. It is an ancient herbal remedy, especially good for babies and young children for expelling wind, or curing hiccups and stomach spasms. As a nerve-soothing tea it is excellent for young and old.

Use. Pain relief — pains of all kinds, but especially those associated with digestion, menstruation. To cure spasms in colic, whooping-cough, hiccups. To expel wind and intestinal gas.

Dose. Make a Standard brew of the leaf sprays and flowers and take a wineglass morning and night. Infants: a teaspoon of the Standard brew, before meals: sweeten with honey.

CAYENNE PEPPER (*Capsicum annuum*. Solanaceae). Except in Africa and South America where it grows wild, it is usually a garden plant under cultivation. Its name comes from the Greek word *Kapto* — I bite, for it is a biting herb with 'fire' in its pods. It has oval, shiny green leaves, and drooping small white flowers which form green pods, which turn red when ripe.

I first learnt its use from the Mexican Indians, who use Cayenne pepper as an internal disinfectant, to overcome the dangers of impure food. The Indians, often having to eat unclean food, suffer no ill effects because they sprinkle powdered cayenne peppers freely as a condiment on most of their eatables. I was able to risk raw milk daily for my children, even from cows and goats of uncertain health, as I cut half a pod of cayenne into every cup of milk and let it steep. That I knew would destroy harmful bacteria. The pepper gave the milk a hot biting taste, but my children learnt to take it with pleasure. I think that this treatment is far better than the harmful pasteurizing of milk which destroys the sensitive life-giving powers. There are no exact measures, as pepper plants themselves differ in strength, so add as much pepper as the drinker of the milk can tolerate without the mouth and throat burning too fiercely. The burning sensation of cayenne pepper is beneficial, never harmful, and soon passes off. I also learnt to use the dried powdered peppers as fumigation against insect pests and rodents when living in primitive places where such things are found in human dwellings.

Cayenne pepper, because it is antispasmodic as well as intensely stimulating, has earned a reputation for giving relief in heart attacks. It is an ancient cure for all types of fevers, and has been used for such treatments by the American and Mexican Indians and African natives throughout their history, and is still in use today.

Use. As a supreme and harmless internal disinfectant. To expel worms. A tonic for all organs of the body, including the heart. For treatment of rheumatism, arthritis, also jaundice and Berger's paraesthesia. Sprinkled freely inside the socks, the pepper will warm the chilled feet of Berger patients. Can likewise be used against frostbite.

To increase fertility and defer senility. For treatment of seriously infected wounds. For fumigation. In ancient times such fumigation was considered a protection against vampires and werewolves.

Dose. A half or whole teaspoon in a large cupful of tepid water — there is no specific dose. Take as much as can be tolerated, fasting, morning and night, i.e. at least one hour before and after meals. At one time, and I have no record of the degree of success achieved, it was said that in heart attacks, a large pinch should be sprinkled frequently on the tongue. I cannot emphasize too often the point I have already made: that when we know that modern resources have made some of these ancient remedies sound not only futile but almost cynically dangerous, it is still worth mentioning them for the sake of the germ of truth contained. It is as foolish to contend that no advance has been made on old herbal lore as to turn a blind eye on those herbal ingredients which no synthetic product can fully replace. Externally: for severe wounds and old sores, disinfect by covering the place with the powdered pepper. It will burn and smart for a brief time in the way that lemon juice does when applied to wounds, but likewise is harmless and highly curative.

For fumigation, sprinkle several tablespoonfuls of the powdered pepper on a tin lid, place it over a slow flame, seal up all the shed or room and allow the pepper to fume until all burnt up. Renew several times if necessary. Cayenne is a pungent fumigator detested by vermin, but it is not poisonous in any way, and any place treated with cayenne can be used very soon after fumigation.

CELANDINE (Greater) (*Chelidonium majus*. Papaveraceae). Found in waste-places, amongst rubble and on old walls. Its foliage is rather hairy and of yellowish tint, the flowers are small, poppy-shape, bright yellow, and produce horned fruits. The greyish stems when broken yield an acrid orange juice. The plant yields a natural dye. Greater celandine has many internal uses in herbal medicine, but as it possesses slightly poisonous properties I am only advising its *external* use in treatment of eye ailments and warts, for which this herb is rightly famed.

Use. To make a soothing and healing eye lotion, boil two dessertspoons of cut herb — including the flowers when possible — in one pint of water. When cold, add one part of the herb brew to one part of raw milk, and bathe the eyes in this. Bathe the eyes thrice daily. For warts: use the raw juice pressed from the main stems, and rubbed directly on to the warts. Renew three times daily.

LESSER CELANDINE (*Ficaria verna*. Ranunculaceae). Known also as Pilewort, it has nothing in common with the greater Celandine, except in being also a medicinal herb. Found in marshy places and by sides of rivers and streams. Leaves heart-shaped, shiny, flowers starry and glossy, bright yellow. A low-growing plant. A salve made from the pulped raw leaves rubbed into cold cream or lanolin, and applied to piles, gatherings, swellings, gives much relief and will often cure the trouble.

CELERY (*Apium graveolens*. Umbelliferae). Wild celery, from which the garden celery is developed, likes damp places by sea or river, or marshland, but it will also seed itself in rich soil in gardens. *Apium* was the Latin name for either wild parsley or wild celery. Its leaves are somewhat similar to those of common parsley, but much wider, and the whole plant is much taller. Flowers are in umbels, small, white to yellow. The whole plant has a strong pungent, biting scent, from the oil — *apiol* — found principally in its leaves. This herb is one of the best for prevention and cure of all forms of rheumatic ailments, also for neuralgia. A remedy for liver trouble, dropsy, tumours. Removes stomach gas, will restore appetite: especially good for children in this respect. The whole plant is used, root to seed.

Use. In rheumatism, arthritis, sciatica, neuralgia, all liver ailments, including jaundice. Will cure swollen stomach in adults and children. Restores appetite to old and young. Will steady the nerves, ease high blood-pressure, improve eyesight.

51

Dose. Eat daily as much as possible of the raw stems, grated raw roots, grated raw leaves, and take the powdered seeds as 'celery salt' (not the same as celery-flavoured salt). The seed is rich in natural soda and is therefore a valuable tonic. Use the powdered seed in larger amounts than you would common table-salt.

CENTAURY (*Enythroea centaurium*. Gentianaceae). (Listed also as *Centauria umbellatum* or *Centauria vulgare*.) Found in fields and hilly places and on sea-cliffs. Leaves are tiny and narrow, the lower ones in a rosette; flowers are star-shaped and pale pink, occasionally red. The whole plant is very bitter. It is one of the best of the bitter tonics and is highly prized by the American Indians. A remedy for ailments of blood and liver. Externally it is used for wound treatment and to deter mosquitoes.

Use. Treatment of jaundice, enlarged liver, biliousness. Blood impurities, eczema. Externally as a lotion for all types of sores and wounds and to cleanse sore mouths and to cool inflamed gums.

Dose. A Standard brew of the whole herb. Take two tablespoons before meals. Use the brew freely for external use, pouring on to wounds, as a rinse for mouth and gums.

CHAMOMILE (*Anthemis nobilis*. Compositae). Found in waste places and as a garden weed. Leaves are feathery, flowers are small, white, daisy-form with yellow centres. It is a very fragrant herb, of sweet apple scent. The flowers yield an oil much used by Arab herbalists. It is one of the best remedies for infants' ailments, being tonic and soothing, and is recognized by the orthodox medical profession as a valuable medicine for the young, especially in France and Spain where numerous doctors prescribe it. Equally useful for female ailments. Used in the treatment of ulcers, tumours, lassitude due to congestion and poor body tone. The brew of dried or fresh flowers is particularly useful as a febrifuge. And to cure insomnia and depression.

Incidentally, chamomile may be planted to replace grass seed or turves where drought conditions prevent a lawn from

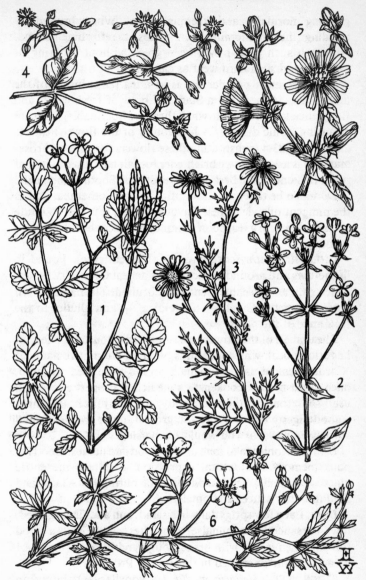

Plate 3. 1. Celandine (Greater) 2. Centaury 3. Chamomile
4. Chickweed   5. Chicory 6. Cinquefoil

growing normally and keeping green. When bruised by treading the chamomile lawn yields a refreshing aroma. Although such a lawn will keep green without watering, it cannot stand such hard wear as can grass.

Use. The most popular use is as a tea (an infusion of the dried leaves is used, but a Standard brew of fresh leaves and flower heads is preferable when these are obtainable. Both are cleansing, tonic drinks). A hair lotion of the flower heads is made, pp. 183-4 (substituting these flowers for sage and rosemary). It is a well-known brightener for fair hair, used as a final rinse. It is one of the best of all eye lotions. Soothes and heals.

Dose. To be taken by the cupful, like any other tea, and as the pungent oils yield their flavour readily, it is best to dilute and sweeten with a teaspoon of honey per cup when the patient is young.

CHERVIL (*Anthriscus sylvestris*. Umbelliferae). Found in hedgerows and around gardens. Has delicate, feathery leaves, which emit an agreeable scent when bruised. The name chervil comes from the Greek — 'to rejoice' — and alludes to the fragrance of the plant.

The umbels of the flowers are small and colourless. The fruit has a long beak which gives this plant an alternative name of 'Garden beaked-parsley'. This is an old-fashioned pot herb, once much used in cookery: its medicinal properties are also useful as it tones up the whole body, especially the brain, and is a good digestive remedy. If you grow it, make frequent small sowings in rows, as you would for parsley.

Use. As a tonic tea to tone up the blood and nerves. Good for poor memory and mental depression. Sweetens the entire digestive system. Well-known as a flavouring for salads, and used in butter sauces and omelettes.

Dose. Eat a few sprigs daily in a salad, and add finely grated, raw, to sauces, mayonnaise, omelettes, etc. Gives a good flavour when mixed with bread dough and baked in loaves of bread — sometimes used in this way in Provence.

CHICKWEED (*Stellaria media*. Caryopyllaceae). Found in fields and ploughed land. Usually indicates a rich soil. Leaves are small, soft and rather yellowish. Flowers are tiny, and held within green bracts. It has a good taste and therefore can be eaten freely in salads when it is still young, before it turns stringy. This is one of the few wild herbs, rich in copper and iron, which is palatable. This small herb, often classed as a troublesome weed, is one of the supreme healers of the herbal kingdom and has given me wonderful results. It is equally beneficial used externally and internally, and fortunately is almost evergreen, growing well in mid-winter and continuing into the late summer. It is a healing demulcent, and possesses remarkable drawing powers, absorbing quantities of impurities when applied to the skin. This small herb possesses many of the healing properties of that famed remedy of the American Indians, Slippery elm tree bark.

Use. As a soothing and healing agent for the whole digestive system, to cure ulcers of stomach and elsewhere. For all internal inflammation, from bowels to lungs. For colitis.

For irritations of the genitals. For cure of all types of skin sores, including erysipelas. For such eye ailments as ulcers and styes. Eaten as a salad improves the eyesight.

Dose. A handful eaten raw twice daily, chopped fine into a salad. Or make a Standard brew and drink a small cupful three times daily, before meals. Externally the herb can be applied as a lotion for skin and eye eruptions. The best skin application is the fresh herb, washed, and then applied directly on the wound, sore or ulcer, holding in place by covering with larger washed leaves, such as cabbage, lettuce or geranium, and then binding with cotton bandages. Change the chickweed every three hours or so, applying fresh. The chickweed will be found very hot, and drenched with the impurities it has drawn out from the skin tissues after each application.

CHICORY (*Cichorium intybus*. Compositae). Found in pastures and on bank-sides. Likes a rich soil for it is very deep-rooting. Leaves are small, greyish, oval. Stems (and root) are tough. Flowers are strap-petalled, wheel-shape, and of a beautiful blue, and very numerous. The long taproot of this plant contains many of its excellent medicinal properties. This plant is an important tonic herb. Bitter-tasting as it is, it is quite edible. The long roots tap the lower mineral layers of the soil and are eaten as well as the leaves. These roots, gently roasted and then ground, are a well-known substitute for, or a mixture with, coffee. The roots are also eaten boiled and are a popular food with Arab villagers. This herb takes its name from the Arabic, *Chicouryeh*. The whole plant is a valuable digestive and nerve tonic. 'Witloof' is the garden variety, grown for its roots rather than its salad leaves.

Use. Tonic and nervine and an excellent remedy for jaundice and all liver disorders. Also for anaemia, weak sight, infertility. Will restore appetite and tone up the entire digestive system, and strengthen the digestive juices.

Dose. Eat as many as possible of the young leaves, fresh, natural, or blanched, in a daily salad. A half-dozen of the flowers can also be eaten. The older leaves can be eaten lightly boiled, as can the roots. The roots, roasted and ground, can be used as a beverage instead of coffee, and they possess superior health properties and no harmful drugging elements (see also recipe for Dandelion coffee under DANDELION, on page 67).

CHIVES (*Allium schoenoprasum*. Liliaceae). Known also as Chive-garlic. Found in damp meadows. Leaves grass-like. The plant's name means rush-leaved onion. It only grows a few inches high, bears round, onion-type balls of purple flowers. Chives possess all the pungent, antiseptic powers of onions in a mild form, and are one of the best means of giving onion elements to infants. For adults chop up in cream cheese, sprinkle on potatoes.

Use. A general tonic and blood-cleanser. Improves appetite.

Dose. A spoonful of the leaves chopped fine with salad or between bread slices, once or twice a day.

CINQUEFOIL (*Potentilla canadensis*. Rosaceae). Found on waste land and along roadsides. Leaves are of attractive silver colour, five-fingered, of palm-tree form. Flowers single, yellow, flattish, and four-petalled. This herb is not much used, which is a pity, for it is very powerful. It is seldom mentioned in herbals, yet its botanical name is from the word *potens* (powerful), alluding to its medicinal powers. It is a nerve sedative and a general astringent. I value this herb very much.

Use. Epilepsy and all hysterical disorders. As a wash for wounds of all kinds, and for sore mouth or gums, as a gargle for inflamed or ulcerated throats. To be syringed into the nostrils to cure sinus infections.

Dose. Infuse a large handful in a pint bottle of white wine and take a wineglassful morning and evening.

CLEAVERS (*Galium aparine.* Rubiaceae). A climbing plant found in hedgerows and fields where there are bushes. Small leaves and tiny, almost colourless flowers which are succeeded by small, prickly, ball-shaped fruits. This 'goose-grass' is notable for its hairy stems, armed with hooked bristles which cling to other vegetation and to passing animals. Cleavers are rich in minerals, and especially rich in silica which exerts a powerful influence on hair and teeth. It is refrigerant, laxative and tonic and is much used in diseases of the urinary system. Its refrigerant properties make it excellent for fever treatment and for skin troubles, including dandruff. It is also an effective jaundice remedy. Taken internally as a hair tonic and to check tooth decay. An old-time farm-workers' tonic added to beer. Externally a great poultice to reduce tumours, and is used for skin cancer.

Use. All fevers including smallpox and typhus. Treatment of bladder and kidney ailments, including stone and gravel, inflammation of the kidneys, suppression of urine, scalding urine. For all skin disorders, including cancer. An old remedy for scrofula, although of course the reduction of scrofular swellings is only a small part of the story, with scrofula sometimes indicating phthisis. Derangement of liver and gall-bladder. Rheumatism, arthritis, dropsy. Externally as a poultice for abscesses, tumours, cysts. As a lotion to cleanse the complexion of acne and other impurities. As an under-arm lotion to neutralize acid perspiration.

Dose. A handful of the herb, pounded small and infused in milk. Take two tablespoons before meals. Or make an infusion by macerating a large handful of the plant in a half pint of near

57

boiling water, keep the water warm for half an hour, then drink the resulting brew. A small cupful before meals. Or cleavers can be eaten as spinach. Not very palatable, but tolerable.

CLOVER (red) (*Trifolium pratense*. Leguminosae). Found in pastures and gardens. Leaves are trefoil shape, sometimes mottled with paler shade. Flowers are in red globes, and are richly honey-scented. Considered by herbalists as being a God-given remedy, it is one of the few herbs which are known to exert a beneficial influence on cancer of all types, and success has been recorded by herbalists, especially in America. Often called 'the prize herb', it is much valued for its alkaline property. A pleasant-tasting herb, it is beneficial to young and old and helps in a long list of ailments, whether mild or chronic. It is useless to try and list them. But is especially good for cleansing the blood, soothing the nerves, promoting sleep, and restoring fertility.

Use. As given above.

Dose. The flowers are used. A small amount may be eaten raw, shredded into a salad. Make Red Clover tea, by infusing a heaped dessertspoonful of the flowers in water just off the boil, allow to steep well and then sweeten with honey. Or make a Standard brew for medicinal treatments, and take a small cupful before meals.

CLOVER (white) (*Trifolium repens*. Leguminosae). Found frequently in meadows and pastures. Leaves similar to those of red clover, but bigger than the red clover, and the flowers are white to cream and very richly honey-scented. This is an old-fashioned but well-proved blood-cleansing herb, also of value externally to heal old sores.

Use. Similar to red clover, only not so powerful and has not been known to give any effective results in cancer treatment.

COLTSFOOT (*Tussilago farfara*. Compositae). Found on banks and waste places. One of the earliest flowers of the European springtime. The flowers appear before the leaves. The leaves, almost round, paler on underside and with thick downy 'web' on upper surface; they are rather fragrant and retain their scent after drying. The flowers are wheel-form of bright yellow and richly honey-scented. The stems are scaly. The name *Tussilago* is derived from the power of this plant to banish coughs. Indeed it is one of the supreme pectoral herbs. It is also a good poultice herb. The whole plant is medicinal.

Use. Cure of coughs, pneumonia, pleurisy, bronchitis, asthma, tuberculosis: gives great relief in whooping-cough and spasmodic cough. Will expel mucus from throat and lungs. It is also a useful fever herb; the peasants say that it comes in time for the spring fevers. Externally, the pounded leaves make a good poultice. Popular amongst gypsies as a 'tobacco' (the dried leaves).

Dose. Make a Standard brew and take a wineglassful three times daily. In coughs take spoonfuls sweetened with honey, every few hours. Use the dried, powdered, leaves as you would use snuff, sniffing up the nostrils to remove obstructions of the nasal passages and relieve sinus infections. Externally, pounded fresh leaves are applied as a poultice to swellings and inflammations. The leaves can also be applied to the lung area as an external pack; or soak cotton in the Standard brew of the leaves and apply hot to the pulmonary region.

COMFREY (*Symphytum officinale*. Boraginaceae). Found in damp places, by ditches, etc. Its leaves are oval and rough, flowers are pale blue-pink, bell-form and borne in drooping clusters. Sometimes they are yellowish. The borage family of plants is a wonderful one in herbal medicine, and comfrey is the greatest of the group. I think so highly of this plant that I have taken the trouble to import plants from England for cultivation in my garden in Galilee. It is, indeed, another of the small company of 'wonder' herbs, being good for almost every ill of mankind. Comfrey's greatest repute is for its peculiar powers upon the bones and ligaments. It has the power to aid the speedy knitting together of fractured bone ends, hence its country name of 'Knit-bone'. The leaves, stems and roots are the parts used.

Use. To aid the knitting of fractures and broken bones, to strengthen strained or weak ligaments and muscles. Also a remedy for rheumatism, arthritis and allied ailments. Its mucilaginous content, especially rich in the root, makes comfrey an important remedy for all disorders of the lungs, including tuberculosis. For treatment of internal ulcers, also externally ruptures and protruding navel and infections of the navel. Externally the leaves make a valued poultice for all types of bruises, swellings and sprains. Also old sores including gangrenous forms, and for burns, whitlows, thorns and splinters in the flesh. Also as an insecticide, the fresh leaves used as a rub.

Dose. Eat three or four medium-sized leaves twice daily (the leaves are rough to the mouth and somewhat bitter, but tolerably palatable). Or the leaves can be cut small and mixed into salad or a dish of potatoes (leaves to be uncooked). Or a Standard brew can be made and a cupful taken before meals. For external use, a cotton cloth can be wrung in the heated brew, when quite hot, and applied to the ailing parts. A poultice is made of the fresh leaves: pulp them first to reduce their roughness and then bind where required, layering them inside a fine cotton-wool pad. A pack of the fresh leaves is prepared as above on account of their roughness, and is applied to the navel, held in place with bandages soaked also in comfrey brew. The well-bruised roots can be used instead of the leaves, or with the leaves. You can rub the leaves on a grater and add to sour milk as a vitamin-rich tonic.

CORIANDER (*Coriandrum sativum*. Umbelliferae). Found in fields and around gardens. Leaves are dark green and fan-like, rather broad for a member of the Umbelliferae. Flowers, small, in umbels, pinkish white in colour. Its leaves have a peculiar rather fetid scent when bruised, and the plant is related to a word meaning 'bug'. Misnamed! I find its odour agreeable.

The leaves are much used as a tonic flavouring herb, especially in South America and China. It is sometimes called 'Chinese parsley'. As well as being an important stomach remedy it is also very strengthening to the heart. The leaves and seeds are used to improve the taste of other herbs when these are not palatable.

Use. A tonic for stomach and heart. To cure chronic indigestion, griping pains in the stomach and bowels, pains in childbirth.

Dose. Three or four sprays of leaves, eaten raw as a salad herb, or a half-teaspoon of the seeds, mixed with honey and eaten raw, before meals; or make a tea from the seeds, and drink several tablespoons of it, sweetened with honey, before meals.

CORN (Indian Corn or Guinea wheat) (*Zea mays*. Graminaceae). Found in pastures and on hill slopes (also widely cultivated), being one of the most important cereals of mankind. Leaves grass-form but very broad and shining. Flowers are white and feathery, both male and female. The cobs formed from the female are well known, and have many medicinal uses as well as providing a valued and much-used cereal food for men and animals. Corn is the only known cereal which alone can sustain life, without other food, over a long period. Dieticians say that the superb teeth and hair of the Mexicans are due to their basic diet of corn. Corn contains a rich oil as well as high quality starch, minerals and vitamins. Also sugar milk for strengthening the bones and as a liver tonic. The leaves of the cob and the inner 'silk' are all medicinal. The 'grains' when young resemble human teeth.

Use. As a food for young and old. Corn-meal (whole grain) makes an excellent addition to milk as a food for infants. The kernels when young should be eaten raw off the cob — in that form mankind obtains a supreme and good-tasting health food. Corn-meal can be cooked like rice, using a little corn oil and the appropriate amount of cold water. The traditional flavouring is garlic and cayenne peppers. The leaves (the inner tender ones) bound over wounds and sores promote healing and draw out offensive matter. The silk, found in the cobs wound around the kernels, is one of the most useful remedies for all ailments of kidneys and bladder. It sooths troubles of the prostrate gland (used internally and externally on the genitals), and it is said to be a remedy against bed-wetting in infants. The silk can be eaten — and some *should* be — raw when fresh, or make a tea, using one tablespoon of the

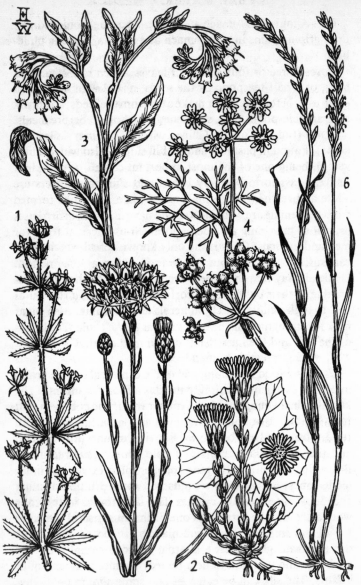

Plate 4. 1. Cleavers 2. Coltsfoot 3. Comfrey
4. Coriander 5. Cornflower 6. Couch Grass

fresh silk or a half-tablespoon of the dried, to one cup of water, and make as a Standard brew. Sweeten with molasses preferably. Externally the fresh (or the soaked dried) silk can be applied as a poultice. Good for drawing pus from boils and old or infected wounds. Applied as a thick pack and bound into place with a wet cloth.

Note. Corn cobs dry up very quickly when gathered, and then it is no longer possible to eat them raw, which is the most healthful way. I have found a method of prolonging their freshness for a full week. Merely stand the gathered cobs in a shallow dish of cold water, their stems, at the base of the cobs, in the water and keep the cobs well shaded by hooding over with brown-paper bags, to exclude all light. Stand them in a cool place.

CORNFLOWER (*Centaurea cyanus*. Compositae). Found in cornfields. Has narrow leaves and brilliant, thistle-form, blue flowers. Its nervine powers are highly rated by herbalists. A proven eye remedy, helpful in many forms of non-structural eye disorders, from weak sight to chronic inflammation and corneal ulcers.

Use. As a tea to soothe and cure the nervous system, a remedy in certain forms of temporary paralysis, also for nervous indigestion. Externally for treatment of eye ailments, insect bites including that of the scorpion, and wounds.

Dose. A few flowers can be eaten raw in a salad: also make a tea of the flowers, and take a cup twice daily. Improved with the addition of aromatic herbs such as rosemary, thyme, etc.

COUCH GRASS or TWITCH (*Agropyron repens*. Graminaceae). Found on waste land and in pastures and gardens, where it is considered a most troublesome weed. Its leaves are long, coarse and very tough, its roots are runner form, white and fleshy and jointed, flower spikes are brownish. A herb known for its beneficial effects on the urinary system, also a good spring tonic. Dogs eat this grass with relish to cleanse themselves through mouth and bowels, so it is often called 'Dog grass'. Cats also use it.

Use. Urinary ailments, including inflammation of kidneys

63

and bladder, stone in bladder, gravel. Also jaundice, gall-stones, constipation. Is a kidney and bladder cure.

Dose. The leaves can be boiled quickly (like spinach) and eaten: they will have to be well chewed as they are tough. Or a strong Standard brew may be made from the roots, a heaped tablespoonful of the roots cut into small pieces, to one and half cups of water. Bring the cold water to the boil, simmer for three minutes, allow to steep well, and take in cupfuls, sweetened with honey or molasses, one cup morning and night.

COWSLIP (*Primula veris*. Primulaceae). Found in meadows and sunny slopes. Likes chalky soils. Leaves are pale and long, oval, flowers are graceful and drooping, bright yellow and of small, primrose form, in pale calyces, very richly honey-scented. A favourite gypsy herb. Makes a good nerve tonic tea as well as a powerful medicine. Its properties are nervine, this herb being extremely calming to the nervous system.

Use. For nervous ailments, including headache, hysteria, fits, sleeplessness. Chorea and epilepsy. To induce sleep when pain is present. In a concentrated form, cowslip is an anaesthetic.

Dose. Six to eight flower heads eaten with salad, twice daily. Or make a Standard brew from the flower heads, and take a small cupful, morning and night, sweetened with honey.

CRAB-APPLE (*Pyrus malus*. Rosaceae). Found in woods and hedges as a small shrub. Has narrow oval leaves with deep-cut edges. Flowers are small, stalked, white and fragrant, in clusters, flowering in early spring. Fruits are small, round, red or yellow and are the origin of the domestic apple, the name being *abhall* in Gaelic. From crab-apples was made the old-fashioned and potent 'magic' drink, verjuice.

Use. Tonic and cleansing, anti-scabies. A cure for all stomach and bowel disorders and for diarrhoea.

Dose. Eaten as a fruit. A half cupful. For diarrhoea, it is taken pulped, scalded with hot (not boiling) water. In half cupful doses, three times daily, sweetened lightly with honey.

CRANESBILL (*Geranium maculatum*. Geraniaceae). Found in hedgerows and near woodlands. Leaves are rounded with scalloped edges, plants are small, purple-pink, of geranium form. The fruits have a long barb, like the beak of a crane, hence its common name. The root is highly medicinal, being a powerful astringent, both for internal and external use. As an astringent it has few equals, in fact.

Use. Treatment of dysentery, diarrhoea, colitis. Also mouth and throat infections, wounds, haemorrhages, indeed wherever a powerful astringent is needed, either internally or externally. Also used to stop undue bleeding after extraction of teeth, sprinkling the bleeding area with the dried, powdered root. A cranesbill root is mild and free from unpleasant taste and so can be given to infants and invalids without difficulty.

Dose. A dessertspoonful of the powdered root to a cupful of water, morning and night. Or make a Standard brew from similar measures, a dessertspoonful to a cupful of water, and take two tablespoonsful of the brew three times daily before meals.

CURRANT (Black) (*Ribes nigrum*. Saxifragaceae). Found wild in woodlands, cultivated in gardens. Foliage is rose-like and possesses a pungent scent, flowers are small, whitish, forming clusters of very juicy, purple-black berries. The fruit is cooling (refrigerant) and soothing, also nervine. It is especially used by herbalists for its beneficial action upon mouth and throat. Because of this property the fruit is often known as 'Quinsy berry'.

Use. Cure for oral and throat ailments, to strengthen the gums. Treatment of fevers, especially in infants. To cure anaemia, prevent miscarriage, and for most disorders of pregnancy. A dysentery remedy, a good vitamin source.

Dose. In fevers and throat ailments give a wineglassful of the juice pressed from the fresh berries every three hours if possible. Or make a Standard brew from the leaves. The fresh juice is preferable. Against miscarriage, eat freely of the berries; when not available take a morning cupful of a brew of the leaves. Blackcurrant purée is sometimes available in cans or jars from good-class chemists.

CURRANT (Red) (*Ribes rubrum*. Saxifragaceae). Similar to Black Currant in type and medicinal virtues. Although this bush-plant is called Red Currant, the fruits are often white, especially in the wild state. Although more powerfully laxative and refrigerant than the black species, it does not possess the same strong curative powers for throat and mouth and the female genital organs.

Use. All fevers, constipation, jaundice and all liver disorders; vermifuge.

Dose. One cupful of the berries twice daily. Or a Standard brew of the leaves, a cupful every morning, or more frequently for jaundice and liver disorders.

DAISY (*Bellis perennis*. Compositae). Found in fields, woodlands, gardens. Leaves are oval, growing in rosettes on the ground, flowers are round, white, many petalled, sometimes pink-tipped. A very well-known plant. Celebrated as a wound herb. The leaves are the medicinal part.

Use. External and internal. Treatment of skin disorders, wounds, bruises. To cleanse the nasal passages.

Dose. Some of the smallest leaves, when young, can be eaten raw in salad. Make a Standard brew of the leaves, large or small, and take two tablespoons three times daily. Use also the brew as a lotion for wounds. Pound up the leaves to a pulp and stir into melted cold cream or butter, and use as a salve: add a pinch of cayenne pepper to every teaspoonful of the salve before it hardens, to make it more effective. For nasal treatment, steam the leaves, roll into pellets and push up the nostrils as far as possible. Keep there for as long as the insertion can be tolerated.

DANDELION (*Taraxacum officinalis*. Compositae). Found on open land, in meadows, and along waysides. Leaves long, tooth-dented, flowers daisy-form, bright yellow, heavily honey-scented, later forming white, fluffy 'clocks'. The leaves and stem exude a white juice when pressed. This is one of the most esteemed plants of the herbalist, a favourite of the great Arabian herbalist Avicenna. It is blood-cleansing, blood-tonic, lymph-cleansing. Also has external uses for treatment of warts and hard pimples. American Indians use the split stem for applying by rubbing, to bee stings.

Use. Blood-cleansing, for all disorders of liver and bile (especially jaundice). A diet of the greens improves the enamel of the teeth. Helps in diabetes, obesity, over-sleepiness. The white juice for application to warts, old sores, blisters.

Dose. A half-dozen or so of the leaves eaten daily. Being rather bitter, they should be mixed with some milder salad herb such as lettuce.

Dandelion coffee is made from the roots, which should be collected at the end of the year for this purpose. After careful cleaning, they are oven-dried at a low temperature for several hours, until they emit a pleasant 'roasted' aroma. They are then ground to a fine powder. A little pure coffee may be mixed in with the dandelion root to improve the scent and flavour. Also roasted chicory root can be added, a teaspoon to every twelve teaspoons of dandelion coffee.

DEVIL'S BIT SCABIOUS (*Scabiosa succisa*. Dipsacaceae). Found in meadows and borders of woodland. Leaves are greyish, rather hairy; flowers small, daisy-shape, usually blue, sometimes white, prominent and with many stamens, strongly honey-scented. The root is peculiar in its blunt end, as if cut off abruptly or bitten. Legend says that this plant is so beneficial to mankind that the devil bit a piece off the root hoping to kill the plant. It is especially good for female ailments, also a nervine, and of use in epilepsy and chorea. For the larger Scabious *see* page 147.

Use. Treatment of menstrual irregularities, uterine disorders, vaginitis. Also veneral disease. As a nerve tonic, and in treatment of hysteria, epilepsy, chorea, bad temper.

Dose. A Standard brew of the flowers. Take two dessertspoonsful three times daily.

DILL (*Anethum graveolens*. Umbelliferae). Found in hedgerows. Has feathery, dark green, very aromatic leaves, and umbels of small, yellowish flowers, which produce the well-known half-moons of fragrant brown seeds.

Dill is so well known as a carminative for babies and for 'bringing up wind', that it used to be mentioned in Victorian songs! It is a generally beneficial herb. Very rich in minerals it improves the nerves, hair and finger-nails. A favourite herb of the Russians.

Use. Treatment of all digestive disorders, including windy colic and fermentation. Eases wind in babies. A mild tea of the seed, known as 'dill water', is given to babies before breast feeds to improve their digestion. My children benefited much from dill water. (A teaspoonful of seeds to a wineglassful of hot water — steep and give tepid.) Treatment of diarrhoea, fevers. The leaves and seed added daily to the diet of nursing mothers increase the milk flow. A useful addition to olives, breads, biscuits.

Dose. Add several sprays of leaves to the raw salad. Sprinkle the raw seeds — a small teaspoon — on vegetables, in porridge, etc. Dill water for general use; make a Standard brew, and take several tablespoons before meals. For infants, merely place a teaspoonful of the seeds in a cup of boiling water (wineglass size) and steep. Add honey to sweeten, and give frequently. Dill water is one of the best remedies to end fits of temper due to colic in infants.

DOCK (Red) (*Rumex aquaticus*. Polygonaceae). Found in abundance on waste land and in fields. Leaves are lance-shaped and sparse on the stems. Flowers are pale-green turning red, brown, in whorls. This is a cold herb, supremely blood-cooling both for external and internal use. The leaves and root are used.

Use. For all heating of the blood, for skin impurities. Used in bygone days also in treatment of conditions similar to syphilis and leprosy. Externally the leaves are applied to all inflammations of the skin, all rashes, and for inflamed and swollen breasts. I have found an application of fresh dock leaves a wonderful help in cases of poison-ivy poisoning.

Dose. A Standard brew of the root or leaves. Take two table-spoonsful three times daily. Externally. Select young leaves, bruise them slightly. Lay them on the area to be treated, and bandage in place. Renew every four hours or so, replacing the old leaves with fresh. Dock leaves pounded up and stirred into melted butter or cold cream make a cooling and healing salve

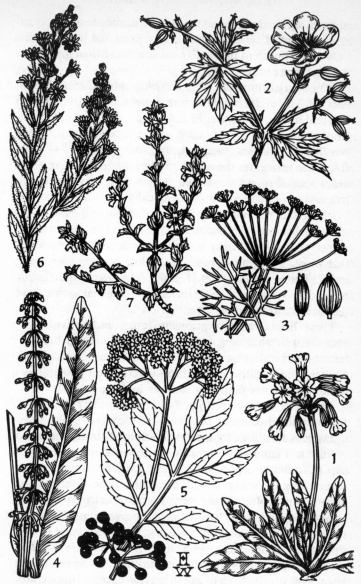

Plate 5. 1. Cowslip 2. Cranesbill 3. Dill (and seed)
4. Dock 5. Elder 6. Elecampane 7. Eyebright

of much value. Dock leaves make good suppositories for treatment of piles. The leaves should be pulped and bound with a little melted soap (a plain olive-oil soap) and then inserted in the anus three times daily.

DOM (Christ-thorn. Jujube. *Zizyphus spina-Christi*. Rhamnaceae). This evergreen shrub sometimes achieves tree-form. It is found in warm climates, in valleys and along coastal plains. Leaves are small, bright, dark green; flowers small, white, woolly, in clusters, very richly honey-scented — their fragrance permeates the air where they are blossoming. Dom bears a small round stone-fruit, which dries very well on the tree and can be stored for many months.

Its flavour is a mixture of those of apple and date. It is a prized delicacy of the Bedouins. The thorns of this shrub are incurving and dig cruelly into the human flesh. Legend says that Christ's crown was made from dom branches, or it may have been a closely related plant, *Paliurus spina-Christi*. Legend also says that the *Christi* name was given to this shrub because Christ loved the dom berries.

These berries are exceptionally tonic, and revive failing appetite, refresh during fatigue from great summer heat, are laxative and vermifuge. I learnt the use of dom berries when in Galilee, and I cultivate this shrub carefully on my land as a tonic food for my family — children and animals.

Use. To refresh and restore. To improve memory. A remedy for high blood-pressure.

Dose. A handful of the berries as desired, fresh or dry.

ELDER (*Sambucus nigra*. Caprifoliaceae). A hedgerow shrub, found also in woodland and gardens. Large broken-form leaves, of strong scent. Flowers are in flat wheel-heads of creamy white colour, waxy, very fragrant, dark purple, edible, strong-tasting berries. This is one of the greatest of all herbs. It is sacred to the gypsies who will not burn it as wood in their fires: they declare that a tree which can help all the ailments of mankind and can restore sight to the blind, is too precious to burn. A favourite herb of the first great doctor, Hippocrates. All parts of the plant are used, from root to berries and bark.

Elder trees survive in the courts of the old synagogues of Safad — ancient town of the mystics of Galilee, birthplace of the Kabala. A magic tree.

Use. The root. The root, washed and soaked, yields a juice valuable in the treatment of lymphatic ailments, and dropsy. Also kidney ailments. Can be used also as a brew; simmer the finely shaved root for several minutes.

The bark. The inner bark, taken from old branches; steep a tablespoonful of the powdered inner layers in a small glass of wine; this is an esteemed remedy against epileptic fits. When the onset of fits is suspected, give a wineglass of the decoction every quarter-hour; give also a wineglassful every night during quiet periods.

The Leaves. A strong Standard brew, strengthened with the addition of geranium leaves and garlic cloves, mixed into the brew, makes a potent skin remedy; will cure itch, ringworm, scrofula. Use internally and externally. Plain elder-leaves brew is a cure for eczema and baby rashes.

The flowers. For colds, coughs and all pulmonary infections. A lotion for all eye ailments. Has restored sight to the blind (when the *nerves* of the eyes were affected by such shocks as bomb blast, etc.). Elder lotion is an old-fashioned but excellent treatment for the complexion and hair. Also for burns and scalds. Good for erysipelas sores. Steep, raw, in water.

The berries. Pounded up in honey, make a soothing and healing remedy for sore throats, coughs. An anaemia remedy, prescribed in tonsilitis and against malignant skin growths (used both internally and externally). The berries are a gentle laxative. Can be applied to burns and scalds.

ELECAMPANE (Lesser) (*Inula viscosa*. Compositae). Found in fields and on hill slopes. Leaves are bright green, rather sticky, of a very pungent scent due to glandular hairs, which protect against grazing flocks. Flowers are bright yellow, starry, small. It is much favoured by the Arabs, who use the leafy sprays in steam baths to cure stiffness of the body and rheumatic complaints. The Spanish peasants hang bunches from ceiling hooks in their homes. The flies gather on the sticky plants which are thrust into sacks at night-time, and the sacks are plunged into water, drowning the flies.

Use. For all ailments of the chest and lungs, including pneumonia, bronchitis, asthma. Also for coughs and hay fever. This herb in vapour and as an internal medicine, warms and strengthens the lungs, and promotes expulsion of mucus from nose and throat. Will soothe coughs and is also a remedy for whooping-cough. Externally, for rheumatism and stiffness. As an insecticide, dried and powdered or as a strong brew.

Dose. Make a Standard brew of the whole herb, take a tablespoon morning and night. Externally, as nasal inhalation, steaming the herb in a kettle and holding the face over the steam, covering head and spout of kettle with a cloth, to retain the aromatic vapours. In steam baths, place a quantity of the herb in the vapour pot or kettle, so that the aromatic oils fill the bathroom and surround the whole body.

EYEBRIGHT (*Euphrasia officinalis.* Scrophulariaceae). Found in meadows and by waysides. Leaves are tiny, in keeping with the whole miniature quality of this plant. Flowers also tiny, white tinged with purple and having a yellow eye. The name of the plant comes from its remarkable power over the eyes; it has restored sight to the blind where blindness resulted from neglected inflammation. The plant is also an astringent and a nerve medicine.

Use. As a lotion for treatment of all eye ailments, including conjunctivitis and ulcers. Also used internally for gastric ailments, and disorders of gall bladder and spleen.

Dose. Externally as a strong lotion: a handful of the whole plant to three-quarters of a pint of water. Bathe several times a day. Also soak cotton swabs in the lotion and place over the eyes, keeping them on for a quarter of an hour or more, adding more lotion to the swabs as they dry up. Also for earache, and as a head pack for headache. Internally a Standard brew, a tablespoonful three times daily.

FENNEL (*Foeniculum officinale.* Umbelliferae). Found on dry banks. It likes coastal regions. Leaves are feathery, very dark green, of pungent scent. Scent is of new-mown hay from which the plant takes its name. Flowers are green-yellow, in umbels. The white hearts of fennel shoots are a prized vegetable, delicious to eat and very healthful. I learnt to use fennel in Algeria and Tunisia, and it is now one of the herbs which I value most.

Use. The leaves, for treatment of all gastric ailments, also constipation, and obesity. Fevers, cramps, rheumatism, diabetes. As a lotion for all eye ailments. Fennel foliage improves memory and is a general tonic for the brain. Externally as a poultice. Hearts of the shoots are a digestive tonic, laxative, and fertility herb.

The roots are not much used, but the Arabs consider them one of the finest of all laxatives. One root taken before meals, twice daily. Grate finely, mix in a tablespoon of bran for improved effect.

The seed, crushed fine and made into a strong tea, speedily expels poison from the blood, therefore should be used after bites from snakes, scorpions, dogs and other animals. Also reduces obesity. Will relieve jaundice.

FENUGREEK (*Trigonella foenum-graecum*. Leguminosae). Found in pastures. Likes sandy soils. Leaves are clover-form, very bright. Flowers are pea-shape, creamy, richly scented. The value of this plant is in its seeds. They are very mineral-rich and nourishing, and in chemical composition they are close to cod-liver oil. The seed is further highly medicinal.

Use. A general tonic and stomach remedy. To increase the body weight.

Dose. A strong tea of the seed (do not strain the tea, eat the seeds also), to strengthen the stomach, intestines, nerves. To give strength to pregnant women, and increase breast milk. A good fever tea, soothing and cooling; add lemon juice and honey. Externally fenugreek seed makes a useful poultice: the ground seed is made into a thick paste with hot milk. Spread on cotton cloth and apply direct upon swellings, abscesses, boils, carbuncles, corns, running sores. As a throat pack, applied hot to relieve soreness. As a throat gargle, use a hot brew.

FERN (Male) (*Aspidium filix mas*. Filices). Found in woodlands and on bank-sides, in shady places. Its leaf shoots are very curled, resembling shepherds' crooks. The fronds are bright green and tall. This is a beautiful and quite common fern. Its distinguishing feature is its root-rhizome, which is the medicinal part, and is large, tufted and scaly. The taste of the root is sickly and bitter-sweet. It contains a green oil, also gum, resin, pectin, tannic acid and albumen: altogether a remarkable rhizome. Through the ages this herb has held its own as a vermifuge; Pliny, Galen, Paracelsus and others of the great herbalists of ancient times, praised it for this quality, especially for its powers to expel tape-worm, and to this present day it is in constant use as a tape-worm remedy, and is sold as a pharmaceutical capsule, proportioned to the age of those for whom it is needed.

Use. A general tonic. Vermifuge, especially against tape-worms of all kinds.

Dose. This remedy is given fasting: the patient should not have eaten food for twenty-four hours and before the male fern dose should take a strong laxative such as castor oil. A doctor or chemist will advise on the amount of oil suited to the age and build of the patient.

The male fern is prepared by slicing finely a piece of root of about six inches in length, which is reduced to a pulp by covering with cold water and then boiling for half an hour. Sweeten the pulp with molasses (which is also a natural laxative) and eat all, together with the water in which it was boiled. A half-hour later, follow with another dose of castor oil. A further half-hour later, take a sloppy meal of soft, flaked oats, liquefied in a little salted, warmed, skimmed, raw milk. Take the same meal later, and nothing else to eat the whole night and day. Then inspect the stool to make sure that the whole worm, *including the head*, has been passed, for the worm can grow again from the head, speedily making new segments to replace those torn away in the treatment, as long as the head remains attached by hooks to the wall of the intestine. Male fern oil capsules, fitted to the age and build of the patient, can be given in hospitals.

FERN (Maidenhair) (*Adiantum capillus-veneris*. Filices).
Found in moist woodlands. Its leaves are frail, many to one
stem, fan-shaped and shimmering and quivering in the wind,
and always brittle. Apart from its fame as a hair tonic, being
used internally and externally to improve the hair, it has other
medicinal powers over heart and lungs.

Use. Treatment for the hair, loss of hair, scanty hair, brittle
hair. Also for chest ailments, cough, and as a heart tonic.

Dose. Make the leaves into a sweet Standard brew, using
honey or brown sugar. Take two dessertspoonsful morning and
night. External use: Standard brew, unsweetened, massaged
well into the scalp every night. Add a few drops of oil of
lavender if possible to the hair lotion.

FERN (Royal) (*Osmunda regalis*. Filices). Found in boggy
places and damp meadowland. Fronds sometimes reach ten
feet or over in height. A vivid green with forked veins.
Considered the most noble of the ferns and named after a
Saxon prince. Its name means both 'peace' and 'mouth-wash'!
The root is the medicinal part, and it is considered to be the
shape of a buck's horn; this gives this beautiful fern the further
name of 'Buckthorn brake'. It contains much mucilage which
it yields to boiling water. Royal-fern Jelly was once a popular
delicacy for invalids, especially for those suffering from wast-
ing diseases. It was given to the young princes of France.

Use. For treatment of coughs and lung ailments, dysentery.
Externally, strengthened with oil of camphor, it is useful for
massage of the spine, in stiff back, stiff neck, and other more
serious ailments of the vertebrae.

Dose. One or two roots, of about six inches in quantity, infused in a pint of hot water. Bring to the boil and then remove
from the heat and steep the fern root. A thick jelly results. This
jelly should be sweetened with honey or brown sugar, and
flavoured with ginger, cinnamon and wine, to taste. For
external use, add two drops of oil of camphor to every
tablespoon of the jelly. In France they also add brandy to the
jelly to increase its powers of penetration into the spinal region.
Roots of the common fern (bracken) are edible and can be

ground and made into bread. The gypsies make use of fern roots in this way (and they are also a favourite food item of badgers!).

FEVERFEW (*Chrysanthemum parthenium.* Composite). Found in waste places. Leaves are feathery and the flowers are white/yellow with pointed centres and daisy (chamomile) form. The plant is very aromatic and has quite a pleasant scent. It is famed as a herb for women, as a tonic and general remedy. It has power over the uterus and ovaries.

Use. Prevention of miscarriage. To help in difficult labour and retention of afterbirth. Female hysteria, female infertility. Externally, the whole herb, crushed into a pulp, makes a good pain-soothing poultice. A useful suppository for treatment of piles.

Dose. Make a Standard brew. Take two tablespoonsful morning and night.

FLAXSEED (Linseed) (*Linum usitatissimum.* Linaceae). Found wild in pastures, but mostly a cultivated crop. Leaves are small and pointed and pale green. The flowers are solitary and of a deep blue. The seed is the part used. Flaxseed (full of oil), is very soothing, bland and tonic. It is a valuable nutritive food as well as a superb poultice for external use. The seed should be carefully prepared by soaking overnight, and draining away the water which contains some irritant properties. The soaked seed can then be mixed raw with other cereals, or lightly cooked.

It heals as it feeds, soothing the throat and entire stomach and intestinal linings. The soaked, ground seed is excellent added to bread and cakes, about two tablespoons of prepared flaxseed to one pound of flour. It improves the digestive qualities of the bread or cakes, and keeps them from speedy drying-out.

Use. Treatment of coughs, sore throats, colds, croup. To build up weakly bodies, enrich the blood, strengthen the nerves. Valuable in pregnancy. Treatment also for pneumonia, pleurisy, bronchitis (as a warm tea, made from one teaspoon of crushed seed to one cup of hot water. Add honey and molasses

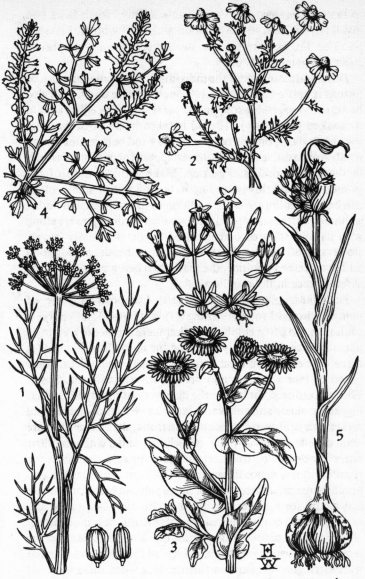

Plate 6.   1. Fennel (and seed)   2. Feverfew 3. Fleabane
4. Fumitory   5. Garlic 6. Gentian

to taste.). Flaxseed *oil* is a valuable laxative for infants and invalids. Will relieve constipation and expel worms. Flaxseed *poultice*. For abscesses, boils, swellings, as a cure for sprains, strained ligaments, bruises.

Dose. Variable, to suit the individual. An average amount of linseed is half a cupful per adult once or twice daily. Can also be added to vegetable soup in the same way as rice (but should be soaked previously). The oil is taken in doses of two teaspoonfuls daily, one before the midday and before the evening meal. As a laxative take two dessertspoonsful or more, fasting, in the early morning. *Poultice*. Make a thick mash of the ground seed, by slowly stirring in boiling water. The poultice can be further improved by addition of other medicinal herbs, as linseed softens them and releases their healing powers along with its own. Grated carrot, shredded parsley, daisy leaves, flowers of St. John's Wort, hops, poppy heads, are all good added to linseed poultice, the mash then being bound over the affected area in the usual way.

FLEABANE (*Erigeron canadensis*. Compositae). One of many herbs used for staunching a flow of blood. Of course it cannot be too often emphasized that there is more to treating a haemorrhage than merely checking the blood loss. Nowadays there would also be treatment for shock, renewal (in some cases) of blood supply, and prompt investigation of causes. The interesting point here is the discovery of the styptic effect. Found on waste and cultivated land. Leaves lance-shaped and rather hairy. Flower heads are numerous, the centre discs are whitish yellow, the ray petals are whitish tinted with pink. The bitter properties of this herb produce an effective wash for repelling fleas, hence its name — fleabane. The plant is also very astringent, and this gives it much value in herbal medicine: it is a cure for summer diarrhoea in children, frequently succeeding when no other remedy proves helpful. It is used internally and as an enema. Also for all intestinal troubles and for internal haemorrhages: haemorrhage of the uterus was treated with astringent fleabane in former days when there were, of course, no facilities for investigating causes.

78

Use. Internally for dysentery, summer diarrhoea, typhus. For internal bleeding, flooding from womb, scalding urine and most bladder troubles, bed-wetting.

Dose. The whole plant is used. The grey down of the seeds can also be used. Make a tea from a dessertspoonful of the cut herb to a half-pint of water, take two dessertspoonfuls of the tea three times daily. In severe dysentery, haemorrhage, etc. take two teaspoons of a stronger brew of tea every two hours. Also give the herb as a warm enema, having steeped a heaped teaspoonful of the herb in a quart of water just off the boil (steeping for half an hour).

FOXGLOVE (*Digitalis purpurea*. Scrophulariaceae). Found in hedgerows, deep ditches, mostly in or near woodland. Leaves are oval and grey, flowers are in tall, attractive spikes and are rose-coloured, freckled with white or brown, and somewhat thimble shaped. From the seed is produced the well-known drug *digitalin*. The whole plant is sedative. Digitalin is a popular drug used as a heart remedy in orthodox medicine, but as it has poisonous properties, I prefer the harmless remedies such as lily-of-the-valley or rosemary. The plant has use as an external remedy, the leaves being the beneficial part, as a sedative. The leaves ease pain, reduce swellings of all kinds, and soothe the twitchings of chorea. Some herbalists maintain that if the *whole* plant is used, the danger of poisoning vanishes.

Use (the leaves externally). To allay pain, inflammations, swellings including tumours, to plug into the ears to soothe earache, to bind over the forehead for headache. A lotion of a small handful of the leaves heated just below boiling point, in one pint of water, makes a soothing eye lotion. Is also a remedy for reducing freckles.

FUMITORY (*Fumaria officinalis*. Fumariaceae). Found along waysides and near hedges. Leaves are fern-like in form and of a greyish colour, flowers are pink-purple, red or yellow, with honey pouches, borne in spikes. The misty appearance of this plant has given it the name of 'earth-smoke'. It is a very esteemed herb and a gypsy favourite. Its chief value is as a cure for all ailments of the liver. As a jaundice remedy, few herbs can excel fumitory. Makes arteries supple. Increases fertility and longevity.

Use. For all ailments of the liver, including jaundice, liver inflammation, enlarged liver. Also to allay biliousness, vomiting, and for general stomach disorders. As a digestive tonic. To cure yawning bouts and inclination to sleep overlong.

Dose. Cut the flowers and leaves small, and infuse a heaped teaspoonful in wine or apple vinegar. One teaspoon of fumitory to every wineglass of wine or vinegar. Infuse for at least twelve hours. Take a half-wineglass morning and night. Externally, apply the infusion in wine or vinegar as a lotion.

GARLIC (*Allium sativum.* Liliaceae). Found in damp pastures and woodlands: also widely cultivated. Its leaves are oval and with very strong onion odour. Flowers are white and starry, also strongly scented. The gypsies worshipped this plant (*moly*) for its remarkable medicinal powers. It is one of the most powerfully antiseptic herbs known to the herbalist. Acts powerfully on the mucous membranes in all parts of the body, and penetrates the blood-stream from the feet to the brain. Vermifuge; expels all toxic elements, kills harmful bacteria. The leaves and flowers are used. To cleanse garlic odour from the breath, chew parsley or mint or basil or thyme, after eating even a little garlic.

Use. Garlic is one of the few herbs found useful in all disorders of the human body. It is further useful when the body is in normal health, as an antiseptic, general tonic and worm deterrent, and in fevers, disorders of blood, lungs — including tuberculosis, for which it is a specific. Against whooping-cough and asthma: for high blood-pressure, goitre and obesity, for rheumatism, arthritis, sciatica. For expelling all kinds of worms, including tape-worms. Protects against all infectious ailments. Also protects the body and hair from parasites. A good external rub in arthritic and rheumatic pains, used hot.

Dose. Preferably take the garlic raw, in the form of a handful of leaves, or two or three cloves, eaten with the salad.

Garlic burns the mouth slightly, but is quite palatable. Or it can be taken in dry, powdered, form, made into pills from three to six grains. Garlic used both externally and internally is a most effective cure for threadworms — so difficult to eradicate. Several cloves are taken night and morning, fasting; at night a raw clove, smeared with oil, is inserted into the anus.

Put garlic cloves (about four to one pound of flour) into bread when baking, also add to vegetables when cooking. In that way garlic supplies food value and its own oil, but for medicinal purposes use raw. The juice has use as a glue component.

GENTIAN (*Gentiana campestris*. Gentianaceae). Found in damp places, such as marshes, by lakesides. Leaves are small, simple, greyish. The flowers are its distinguishing feature, being usually of an intense and beautiful blue, four petalled. There is also a yellow-flowered variety, *Gentiana lutea*; the flowers are bigger. A Greek king, Gentius, who was also a great herbalist, gave this plant its name. The American Indians have long worshipped gentian for its medicinal powers; it is their 'blue blossom' remedy. It is a strong tonic, a good liver remedy. Will ease prolonged vomiting when all other treatments have failed. Neutralizes internal poisons. The root is used. 'Gentian bitter' is a tonic extraction from the roots, also used as stomachic. 'Gentian violet' is an antiseptic tincture. It is the quinine of the poor,

Use. As a general tonic and to purify the blood. For indigestion, biliousness, jaundice, prolonged vomiting, lack of appetite. For nervous disorders, including hysteria. To neutralize all forms of poisons such as that in snake and scorpion and rabid dog bites (used internally and externally). Since there is more to the treatment of dangerous bites than dealing with the immediate symptoms, the patient should obtain skilled advice.

Dose. One ounce of the finely shaved or powdered root (freshly powdered) brewed in one pint of water (Standard method). Sweeten with honey, and preferably add other pleasant-tasting herbs such as mint, basil, lime blossom, to reduce its very bitter taste. Two tablespoons thrice daily before meals. Famed Gentian Tonic wine is two ounces macerated steeped in one litre white wine.

GINGER (*Zingiber officinale*. Zingiberaceae). Ginger is not a wild herb. The root is imported from China and West Africa, and is obtainable in pieces or ground into a fine powder, from pharmacies and groceries. As well as being a valued and popular condiment, ginger is highly medicinal. Its properties are stimulating, warming, aromatic, digestive. Ginger will produce sweating and its penetrative powers will quicken paralysed limbs. Also valuable as addition to other medicines, to lessen nausea and to prevent griping.

Use. A general tonic for nerves and digestive organs. Stimulates digestive juices, expels worms, cures colds, sore throats, diarrhoea, indigestion, nausea. Good for delayed menstruation and for exhaustion during or following childbirth. An important ingredient of senna laxative drink, to prevent the typical griping of senna. Take candied ginger against all forms of travel sickness.

Dose. A piece of the root, about the size of a small hazel nut, may be chewed before meals. Or make ginger tea, from a quarter-teaspoonful of ginger (powdered) to a half-pint of hot water, sweetened with molasses and honey, and with a slice of lemon added. Taken this way as a warm drink, it is helpful in cases of delayed menstruation, and for childbirth pains.

GOLDEN ROD (*Solidago virgaurea*. Compositae). Found on open places and by woodlands. Leaves are narrow, pointed, pale green. Flowers growing in tall rods, of tiny, golden daisy-form flowerets, heavily powdered with pollen. This plant is cultivated in gardens for its glowing beauty, and the garden variety can be used as a medicine. This is a famed wound herb. The Saracens preferred not to go into battle without this herb along with them. The American Indians greatly favour it too. It is a powerful tonic of pleasant taste. Useful against fevers and for treatment of all kinds of wounds: it was valued in the Middle Ages as the gangrene herb, but I for one have not discovered which necrotic condition was implied.

Use. Digestive tonic and remedy for most digestive ailments.

Treatment of jaundice, kidney and bladder ailments. In fevers will promote sweating. Externally for wounds, to staunch bleeding, cleanse infections.

Dose. Make a Standard brew and take two tablespoons morning and night.

GOLDEN SEAL (*Hydrastis canadensis.* Podophyllaceae). Found in damp woodland and marshy areas. Leaves are borne in twos on the stems and are palm-shaped. Flowers are solitary, small, white or rose-shaded. The fruit is red and has the form of a raspberry, giving the plant its further name of Ground Raspberry. The root is the medicinal part. It is of rhizome type, internally has long fibres and is of an intense yellow, which yields a permanent dye. The fresh root is juicy, and this is used for dyeing. Turmeric root is another name for this plant. It is a favourite of the American Indians who considered it virtually a cure-all. A new herb to me, I learnt its use from American Seventh Day Adventists, and I share their view that it cures a wide variety of disorders. The golden powder derived from the root could be added to bread, a small pinch to a half pound of flour (but not when you add garlic, see page 81).

Golden Seal is used as a substitute for quinine, and is most effective and less violent in action. It is much used for erysipelas. An excellent eye remedy. The root is the only medicinal part of which I have knowledge. This is rather a costly herb.

Use. Treatment of malaria and all fevers; there are reports of its successful ancient use in conditions closely resembling meningitis, and smallpox or scarlet fever or typhus. Golden Seal has a powerful healing effect on all mucous surfaces, and is therefore of much value in healing stomach and intestinal ulcerations. Also used to soothe the nasal passages, bronchial tubes, bladder — internally and externally. Used also for sore tonsils, sore gums and mouth, sore eyes. Makes a good tooth tonic, brushed in lotion form upon the teeth and over the gums. For eczema, ringworm and all types of skin infections, golden seal excels most herbs. Used in all infections of the genital organs. Also for diabetes, nausea of pregnancy, including morning sickness.

Dose. A quarter teaspoonful of the dry powder, mixed with honey, to be eaten three times daily, before meals. It is slightly bitter but not too unpleasant. For external use, make a 'lotion' by steeping half a teaspoonful of the powder in a large cup of water just off the boil. Or for wounds, etc. merely sprinkle the dry powder directly on to the wound, then cover with green leaves to hold it — using such leaves as lettuce, geranium, cabbage, etc. — and bind into place. The 'lotion' can also be taken as a tea, sweetened with honey, to allay morning-sickness of pregnancy. A cupful should be taken fasting.

GROUND IVY (*Glechoma hederacea* or *Nepeta hederacea*. Labiatae). Found in woods and hedgerows. Leaves are small and grey, flowers small, pale blue, hooded. The whole plant is of a creeping growth. This small herb is a potent tonic and general stimulant; it acts powerfully upon the uterus.

Use. Digestive tonic and treatment of digestive ailments. As a cough remedy, and for tuberculosis. For treatment of retention of after-birth, and for all glandular infections. Externally as a wash, the plant steeped in boiling water and applied: for ulcers, abscesses, ear and nasal infections and spring rashes.

Dose. A Standard brew. Take a tablespoonful three times daily. For treatment of after-birth pains, a cup of the brew every two hours. For external use, apply the Standard brew as a lotion. Chewed-up in the human mouth this herb was an old remedy of grooms and kennel-men for applying to the inflamed eyes of horses or dogs. Likewise, the gypsies so use it for their children.

GROUNDSEL (*Senecio vulgaris*. Compositae). Found on waste land and in gardens. Leaves are greyish and slightly toothed, flowers small, yellow, tubular-shape, like tiny candles and possessing no ray petals. An important tonic herb, being extremely rich in minerals. The Victorians knew of the high mineral content of groundsel, but fed it regularly to their caged canaries instead of eating it themselves! This herb is quite palatable and I use it raw in salads. But — caution! What I (and the New Forest gypsies, for example) do with groundsel is nowadays severely condemned by such authorities as the National Institute of Medical Herbalists who advise that groundsel and ragwort (*senecio aureus*) should NOT be eaten, as they contain certain alkaloids which damage the liver. Groundsel possesses strong drawing powers as well as antiseptic properties far out of proportion to its small size. Mixed with the herb ground ivy (*Glechoma hederacea*) is makes a poultice of high repute.

Use. In consideration of the views of the National Institute of Medical Herbalists, I shall not recommend groundsel for internal use. Externally for all wounds, inflamed places, infected places, sore nipples, whitlows. For treatment of minor eye ailments, applied raw as an eye pack. It also strengthens weak eyes.

Dose. Merely pulp up the raw herb and apply. An old-fashioned but important poultice is made by bruising fresh groundsel and making a mash with the addition of bread soaked in hot milk.

GYPSYWORT (*Lycopus europaeus*. Labiatae). The Latin name refers to the 'wolf's foot' shape of the leaves. Whereas most of the Labiatae have four stamens in the flowers, *Salvia* and *Lycopus* have only two. The white flowers are small, the plant prefers a light, rich soil.

Use. As for Mint. I have read in a French work that the tonic, stomachic and febrifugal properties of Gypsywort are identical with those of *Eupatorium perfoliatum*, and that some of the properties of Agrimony, especially the power to relieve obstruction of bile, may also be attributed to Gypsywort. At present I am not able to vouch for these claims, and recommend that both for Uses and Dosage it be treated as a member of the Mint family.

HAWTHORN (*Crataegus oxyacantha*. Rosaceae). Found in woods and hedges and on heaths and waste land. Leaves are dark and narrow, with cut edges. The flowers are small, white or pinkish, with many stamens. Borne in clusters and are strongly scented. Supposed to bring fairies into houses. Are unlucky if gathered before the first week of May. Fruits are small, red, hard with hard pips and known as 'haws'. The wood of hawthorn is very hard and therefore an excellent tool wood. The hardness and strength of this shrub gives it its Grecian name for strength.

Use. The leafy buds are eaten as a tonic salad. The country name is 'pepper and salt', as they have that very taste. The flowers are also edible, sprinkled on fruit salads, junkets and custards. The fruits are edible and tonic, eaten raw (though rather astringent in the mouth). They make good conserves and fermented make a strong wine. A poultice of the pulped leaves or fruits has strong drawing powers and country people for ages have used hawthorn for treatment of embedded thorns, splinters and also for whitlows. The fruits are also nervine and helpful in prevention of miscarriage.

Dose. As much as desired in salads. Against miscarriage take four to six fruits. The fruits can be dried and stored.

HEATHER (*Erica* — various. Ericaceae). Found on peaty moorlands and hillsides. Leaves are minute, grey-green, tough; flowers, tiny, bell-form and very richly scented with honey. Indeed heathers scent the air for wide distances around where they grow in their pink-purple stretches. Their heather honey makes them highly tonic, apart from their excellent mineral content. Good for heart and nerves, a tonic for invalids and for those who suffer from mental depression. This plant yields a honey highly valued by those with the knowledge and the palate for distinguishing one honey from another.

Use. General debility, impoverished nerves, mental depression, insomnia. Stomach-ache, lack of appetite. Fertility herb. Scottish Highlanders make a cough remedy from a strong brew of heather flowers and plentiful heather honey added.

Dose. Drink as a tea, sweetened with honey. Infuse three or four flower sprigs, in hot water.

HENBANE (*Hyoscyamus niger*. Solanaceae). Found in waste places, especially around towns and villages: often found growing on old walls and amongst rubble and ruins. The leaves are attractively indented and the flowers are yellow with purplish brown markings. The offensive odour comes from the sticky, hairy leaves mainly. Both leaves and flowers yield the alkaloid drug named hyoscyamine, which is poisonous if misused. This is made use of in pharmaceutical practice for lessening the griping action of certain purgatives. On account of this danger, I prefer to use the herb externally only, but Arab friends have told me that they actually chew it to relieve severe stomach pains, and use the herb a good deal in their homes, so possibly they have an acquired and inherited immunity to the worst effects of the drug. Another name for Henbane is Hog's Bean — this is, in fact, the ancient Greek name used by Dioscorides (*hyos kyamos*).

Many herbalists prefer henbane to opium, as it is less habit-forming and also does not cause constipation through the drugging of the intestinal nerves. It is given when opium cannot be tolerated by severely ill patients. For internal use the seeds are used as they are almost non-poisonous. Pigs eat the seeds freely.

Henbane was so favoured as a narcotic in ancient times that according to Josephus Flavius, the head-dress of the High Priest of the Jews was modelled after this plant, with its funnel-shaped corollas. It was used as a general sedative in former times, long before the discovery of anaesthesia.

Dose and *Use*. (The seeds only, internally, six to eight seeds morning and night.) Spasms of asthma, croup, whooping-cough, chronic cough. As a hypnotic to calm nervous frenzy, fits of rage, uncontrolled weeping. The leaves, externally. To soothe inflamed wounds, glandular swellings — including mumps; to apply to throbbing pulses in wrist and head. To ease toothache (the leaves are chewed and then spat out). Earache: make a Standard lotion of the leaves, drop a teaspoonful of the brew (warm) into both ears — even if only one ear is aching.

HENNA (*Lawsonia inermis*. Lythraceae). Found on hillsides and plains, in shrub-form in Eastern lands. Also cultivated with artificial heat. Leaves are narrow, small, grey-green, and profuse. Flowers also profuse small, creamy white in the *alba*

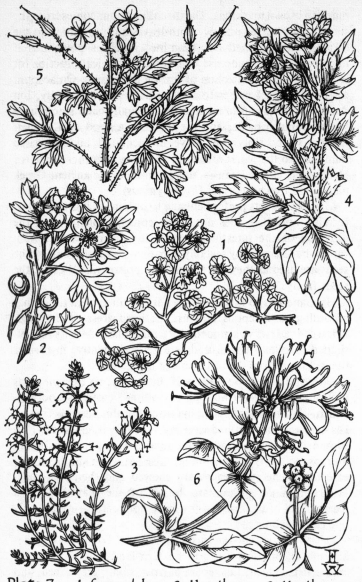

Plate 7. 1. Ground Ivy 2. Hawthorn 3. Heather
4. Henbane 5. Herb Robert 6. Honeysuckle

variety, in rose-pink panicles in the *inermis*, and very fragrant. They give small, blue-black, single berries. The whole shrub, skin of roots, bark of trunk and branches, dried leaves and fresh berries, yield a very popular dye — henna, the *alcanna* of the Arabs. Henna not only tints the hair auburn or black as desired, it is also a hair and scalp tonic. This herb is extremely penetrative and therefore a very effective dye. Its one fault as a hair dye is its astringency and therefore after applications of henna, oil should be rubbed into the hair (preferably a bland oil such as sunflower or corn). As with many astringent herbs, henna is also most cooling, and therefore is used to allay fevers. It is also a useful application to insect bites.

Use. Hair dye (also skin dye: Arabs 'henna' the palms of their hands and the soles of their feet; they find this cooling as well as beautiful). As a head-pack applied upon the head and over the forehead, in headaches and fevers. To draw impurities from the body, by applying to the navel, during high fevers and in jaundice cases. Applied like clay over feet and ankles will reduce swollen feet and soothe aching and burning feet.

Dose. To make a henna pack to dye the hair or soothe the head. Take two cupfuls of henna powder (red or black), stir slowly into this powder one cupful of tepid water — more or less — to make a paste which will not drip off the scalp and hair. Henna pack is further improved by adding one teaspoon of pure vinegar and a half-teaspoon of golden seal root in powder form (see page 83). Heat the mixture slowly, using a double pan. Keep well stirred, and when this is near boiling keep on the flame for a few minutes. Allow to stand and steep for one hour. Then re-heat to blood-heat (as a hair dye) and massage well into the head and hair. Tie a scarf over the head to cover the hair while the henna is working, and to prevent the mixture falling. Leave the henna pack on the hair for seven hours or more, keeping the head covered all the time. Then rinse off, and later apply a little oil to the scalp and hair. For headaches, etc. apply the henna cold.

HERB-ROBERT (*Geranium Robertianum*. Geraniaceae). Found on waste land, in hedgerows and on the outskirts of woods. Greyish in colour, geranium-form leaves, flowers small, pink noticeably scented. This herb is also called Stinking crane's-bill, although it has a rather pleasant, geranium-like aromatic scent. Sometimes the entire plant turns red in the autumn. Like all the geraniums this is a good wound herb, with healing and drawing properties. Internally soothing and antiseptic. A diabetes aid.

Use. Treatment of all forms of haemorrhage, kidney and bladder ailments, tuberculosis, and soothing for some forms of cancer. Externally as a ringworm remedy, and as a wash to remove lice and their eggs. For all kinds of wounds.

Dose. A Standard brew. Take a half-cup morning and night. Externally apply the brew as a lotion. Make an especially strong brew for external use, doubling the quantity of herb to the water used. For wounds apply the leaves, fresh, bruised, and bound into place.

HOLLYHOCK (*Althea rosea*. Malvaceae). Found wild on waste land and rocky slopes. Also widely cultivated in gardens. Leaves are round, large, with hairy undersides of greyish colour. Flowers are large, borne on tall spikes, and have the typical mallow-type square petals. The wild variety usually has rose-coloured flowers. This plant possesses valuable soothing properties. The leaves, lightly boiled, provide a worm remedy suitable for children, one much used by the Bedouin Arabs, wild hollyhock being abundant in many areas where the Bedouins live in their black tents. The leaves, heated in wine, are given to avert threatened miscarriage.

Use. To soothe the digestive tract. To expel worms. Female troubles, inflammation of uterus, uterine tumours, vaginitis, threatened miscarriage. Externally to soothe inflamed flesh, cool the burning of wounds.

Dose. A handful of leaves to half a pint of water or wine. Flavour with a pinch of ginger and cinnamon. Take two tablespoons four times daily. Externally, apply a lotion made from boiling the leaves in water, or apply young leaves, using the upper sides, not the rough undersides, directly on the area to be treated. Or make a poultice of the pulped leaves added to flaxseed mash.

Or make a poultice of the pulped leaves added to flaxseed mash.

HOLY THISTLE (*Silybum marianum*, also *Centaurea benedicta*. Compositae). Known also as Blessed Thistle and Our Lady's Milk Thistle. Found on waste land and by waysides. Leaves are spiky and mottled, of bitter taste. Flowers are purple typically of globose thistle form. This plant gained the name of holy thistle, blessed thistle, on account of its beneficial effects upon all who gather and use it, and for its general usefulness; the root was used as a vegetable, the leaves as a green salad, and the heads as artichokes: all of the plant is edible. It clears the mind of depression and ill humour, and was formerly given to the insane. It is beneficial in ailments of women, and a salad of the young hearts of the leaves, and the stems stripped of their coarse outer cover increases the flow of breast milk. Or a tea of the leaves, Standard brew, can be made for this purpose. Good for all organs of the body, especially the heart and brain.

Use. To purify the blood, cleanse the stomach, liver and kidneys, for heart ailments and as a heart tonic. Treatment of mental depression, suicidal feelings, loss of memory. For women, will regulate faulty menstruation and increase breast-milk.

Dose. A half-handful of the young leaves, trimmed of prickles, or the young stems, eaten once daily. Or a Standard brew of the fresh or dried leaves. A small cupful with honey, morning and night. Eat also the cooked stems and fruits.

HONEYSUCKLE (*Lonicera periclymenum*. Caprifoliaceae). The 'luscious woodbine' found in woodlands and twining in hedgerows. Leaves, oval, shiny, greyish. Flowers spurred, yellow-cream to pale pinky purple, highly fragrant. The whole plant is medicinal. Good for the heart, skin ailments, rheumatic ailments.

Use. All heart troubles and as a heart tonic. Against sore throat, cough, asthma, skin disorders, rheumatism, arthritis and general stiffness of the joints. Swollen glands, dropsy — the bark is used remedially here.

Dose. A small handful of the flowers, eaten raw or made into a tea. Take in the early morning. Or a Standard brew made from one dessertspoonful of flaked bark to a half-pint of water. A French gypsy asthma remedy is a handful of the flowers, well crushed, mixed with sufficient honey and molasses (equal parts) to bind the flowers. Eat a tablespoon of the confection morning and night. Externally, the crushed leaves applied to wounds, sores, ulcers, will promote healing and allay heat.

HOPS (*Humulus lupulus*. Canabinaceae). Found growing on rich, moist land. A hedgerow climber, also widely cultivated. Leaves are vine-form, flowers are of peculiar form, green-yellow, fragrant. The fruit, called strobiles, possess a yellow, resinous dust that is *lupulin*, which gives this herb most of its medicinal virtues. They are pale green, covered with loose scales and are of cone-form. The shoots of hop, blanched and eaten young, are sometimes likened to asparagus. The whole plant is useful for its tonic and therefore nervine properties. It is also pain reducing and hypnotic. It increases breast milk and therefore soothes irritable infants. Hops are known for their use in breweries, but they also are one of the best medicinal plants known to the herbalist.

A favourite plant of the gypsies everywhere.

Use. General tonic. Excellent nervine, sleep inducer, cure for uncontrolled sexual desires and a quarrelsome nature; also for earache, toothache, neuralgia. Will restore poor appetite due to general debility, and its long-term use could prevent anaemia. Worm remover. Externally for aches, wounds, sores, skin rashes.

Dose. If possible, cut the hops small and eat them raw, six to eight flowers morning and night; some honey can be added. Or make a tea from a heaped tablespoonful of hops placed in half a pint of cold water and simmered for two to three minutes. Steep well and drink a small cupful morning and night. Hop pillows were once in popular use — that is pillows made of muslin, and stuffed with hops: to induce sleep, calm the nerves, prevent nightmares. They would be equally beneficial if used nowadays, and would be improved by adding several handfuls of dried lavender flowers to every pillow.

For external use, hop poultices are made from crushed hops worked into a paste with bran, and applied cold, to cure inflammations, swellings, sores, boils, tumours and cysts. A rub for congested lungs or pains in the chest is made from a handful of hops steeped in a half-pint of vinegar or ale, re-heated and used hot.

HOREHOUND (White) (*Marrubium vulgare*. Labiatae). Found in dry, waste places preferring poor soil. Leaves are grey-green, rough, slightly woolly, and have a scent of vines. The flowers are small, white, pungent of scent, and encircle the stems in whorls. This is a bitter aromatic herb. Should be gathered when young, before flowering. This plant contains a powerful substance named *marrubium*. This substance pro-motes perspiration and the flow of urine, and is also laxative and vermifuge. Horehound has long been known as a soothing syrup and tonic candy. Horehound candy used to be on sale in most grocers' shops in Victorian times, and was a favourite with children: a healthful sweetmeat. A well-known throat and lung remedy.

Use. General tonic. Treatment of sore throat, coughs, colds, hoarseness, asthma, tuberculosis and all lung disorders. To reduce fevers, expel worms. Externally for earache.

Dose. Make a Standard brew and take two tablespoons, sweetened with honey twice daily. For earache: drop a half-teaspoon of the Standard brew into the ears several times daily and then massage the base of the ear. To make horehound syrup. Make a syrup from one cupful brown sugar, two table-spoons honey, the juice from half a lemon (about one dessert-spoonful of juice) one teaspoonful soft oil such as sunflower or corn. When the syrup has thickened stir in a large handful of horehound leaves, in the form of a strong brew in water.

Horehound Candy. Into two pounds of brown or lump sugar (the latter is most typical for horehound candy, though less healthful), stir four tablespoons of a strong infusion of dried horehound plant, i.e. the strained liquid obtained from boiling a handful of the herb in one and a half cups of water. Mix one teaspoon of thick honey to every pound of sugar. Boil for a half-hour or more, until a portion taken out hardens when dropped into cold water. Then pour on to a cold marble slab (preferably) or into shallow tin moulds dusted with icing sugar.

HORSE-RADISH (*Cochlearia armoracia*. Cruciferae). Found in waste places and cultivated in gardens. Leaves long, coarse, rough, of biting taste, flowers small, whitish and cross-form. The root-stock is the medicinal part, and is long, with stringy end, white or pink in colour. It has a hot, biting taste, and its 'hot' property makes it a valued remedy for expelling worms, destroying harmful bacteria, and for stimulating the appetite.

Use. A good remedy for urinary troubles. To reduce dropsy and dissolve internal tumours. Externally as a raw poultice, applied to wounds, old sores, swellings and tumours.

Dose. One or two roots daily, taken raw and finely grated. Divide into teaspoon-amounts and take before meals. Eat the horse-radish with bread if its hot pungency cannot be tolerated on the tongue.

HORSETAIL (*Equisetum arvense*. Equisetaceae). Found on waste land and along ditches and roadsides. This plant is of peculiar formation, resembling a horse's tail. The stems are hollow-jointed and the leaves reduced to a mere scale at the points. No flowers are produced, but brown spores are borne on the fertile stems. The high silica content of this plant gives it a hard and quite sharp texture, and peasant people and gypsies put it to use as a pan scourer. It was formerly especially used to scour dairy pails and implements. The plant is highly medicinal, with powerful antiseptic properties, and is a famed vulnerary.

Use. Treatment of stomach and intestinal ulcers, inflammation of the uterus, vagina and bladder (also used externally as a douche). To cure internal wounds of bowels, reduce enlarged anal glands (internal and external treatment). For dysentery, obesity, dropsy. To dissolve stone in bladder (a strong brew). To strengthen hair, finger-nails, enamel of teeth. Externally: for nose-bleeds, laryngitis, ear-pains, toothache, all forms of wounds.

Dose. This is a potent herb. Make a brew from a half-handful of the whole plant to one and a half pints of water (Standard method). Take two dessertspoonfuls morning and night. Externally pulp up the herb, dissolve well in warm vinegar, a handful of herb to a pint of vinegar. For treatment of wounds, dilute the vinegar brew with two parts of raw milk. The whole plant, made into a strong brew, is an effective spray against mildew on roses and vines.

HOUND'S TONGUE (*Cynoglossum officinale.* Boraginaceae). Found on dry banksides and uncultivated land. Leaves are of rough texture and tongue-shaped, thus giving this plant its common English name; they are greyish in colour. Flowers are blue shading to pink, hooded and with funnel. At the base of the funnel is stored nectar; country children like to suck the flowers to take this nectar. I use the flowers, fresh or dried, in herbal teas for table use. The root is the medicinal part, both fresh and dried, but the leaves also are helpful. This is chiefly a poultice herb (and a very effective one), but also has value in treatment of the respiratory system.

Use. Treatment of coughs, excess mucus in nasal passages and throat, congestion and bleeding of lungs, bronchitis. Externally, a poultice from shaved root or bruised leaves, for application to bruises, abrasions, gravel rash, goitre, tumours, burns and scalds.

Dose. A Standard brew of the leaves, or use the shaved root; boil one tablespoonful of root in half a pint of water; allow to stand and brew for several hours, then strain and use. A tablespoon of brew from leaves or root is taken three times daily before meals. Externally, use the bruised leaves applied direct as a poultice, or a cloth soaked in a brew from the root shavings: apply cold.

HOUSELEEK (*Sempervivum tectorum.* Crassulaceae). Found on old rubble, in crevices on roof-tops and walls. Its succulent nature enables it to survive in such arid places. Its leaves are grey-green, in rosettes, and distinguished by their succulence. Flowers are small, rose-coloured, star form, and are borne in spikes. Its use is mostly external for treatment of skin ailments, this being an astringent and very cooling herb. Internally as a vermifuge. The leaves contain lime.

Use. Treatment of itching skin, all rashes, inflammations, erysipelas, burns, warts, stings.

Dose. For worms. Make pills of the pulped plant rolled in flour and bound with a little honey. Take two pills of the plant (pea size), fasting, morning and night. Externally: the pulped plant applied direct to the affected area. For warts, slice leaves in two and apply the moist inner surface to the warts.

HYDRANGEA (*Hydrangea aborescens.* Saxifragacea). Found in woodlands and along banks of streams, also cultivated as a garden plant. Leaves are ovate, dark green, cut edges, large. Flowers are showy, and borne in large corymbs, their colour is white, blue or pink shaded. The bark of the stems peels very freely. This was a favourite of those great herbalists the Cherokee Indians. It is a mild and soothing herb, and is effective in rheumatic troubles and glandular disorders. Also in urinary ailments.

Use. Rheumatism, including its chronic forms. Joint stiffness and paralysis. Bladder and kidney disorders, including stone, inflammation, backache from kidney trouble. Treatment of dropsy and all lymphatic swellings.

Dose. Make a Standard brew from the leaves. Take two dessertspoonfuls morning and night.

HYSSOP (*Hyssopus officinalis.* Labiatae). Found in dry, hilly places. The leaves are long and lance-shaped, and highly aromatic. Flowers are pale blue and hooded, also aromatic, mint-like. This important herb was praised by David in the Bible — 'Purge me with hyssop'. Hyssop is notably successful in relieving catarrh. Some say that the Biblical hyssop was more likely to be the Caper plant. The leaves contain a peculiar yellow oil and sulphur. The whole herb is a great

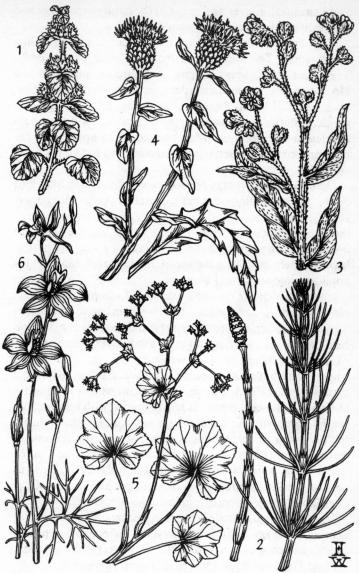

Plate 8. 1. Horehound   2. Horsetail   3. Hound's Tongue
4. Knapweed   5. Lady's Mantle   6. Larkspur

body cleanser, a fever and nerve herb, mildly vermifuge and also valued for the eyes. Regulates the blood.

Use. For all complaints of throat and lungs, including tuberculosis. To expel mucus from all parts of the body. Treatment for asthma, coughs, sore throats, high and low blood-pressure, nervous disorders, including fits and epilepsy. As a remedial lotion for eye ailments, ear ailments and as a gargle. Externally the leaves applied to bruises will allay pain and lessen discoloration. May be used as an application for bites and stings of insects and medusae, and for killing body vermin.

Dose. A few leaves may be eaten raw in salad. As a Standard brew, take two tablespoons before meals: sweeten with honey. As a gargle, if possible add equal parts of sage leaves brew to the Standard brew of hyssop. As a lotion, use the Standard brew. For skin vermin, make a decoction by steeping hyssop leaves, finely cut, in pale ale. Use the same mixture for application to stings and bites.

ICELAND MOSS (*Cetraria Icelandica.* Lichens). This lichen plant is found in damp places. It grows from two to four inches high and is generally brown or grey in colour. It is a dry and cartilaginous moss, drying up to an ash-like substance of grey-white shade. When put into water it swells up rapidly, and when gently boiled and cooled it becomes a fine jelly. This plant is remarkably life-giving and nutritious and will sustain life where little else grows. It is a favourite with reindeer. Its special tonic virtues are due to a substance called *cetarin*, slightly bitter in taste. If it is removed, the moss becomes merely of nutritional value. It is much used in treatment of tuberculosis, which is rather prevalent in Iceland. Used also to nourish weakly children, invalids, aged people. To soothe the intestinal tract in dysentery, and similar ailments.

Use. Treatment of malnutrition and rickets. To give strength to infants, the aged, and for all invalids. Tuberculosis, chronic catarrh and coughs, also bronchitis. Dysentery and diarrhoea.

Dose. One teaspoonful stirred into a cup of water just off the boil. Sweeten with honey or molasses. Or a half-cup of water can be used and then a further half-cup of milk added: sweeten with honey, maple sugar, molasses. Also add a little cinnamon, nutmeg and a pinch of powdered cloves, to make a nutritious milk jelly.

IRIS (*Iris tuberosa*. Iridaceae). Found in damp places and coastal regions. Formerly much cultivated in herb gardens for its medicinal properties: leaves are stalkless, reed-form, flowers pale blue, colour streaked (the very name 'Iris' means rainbow), and sweetly scented. This plant is a mild general tonic for the whole human body, but especially beneficial to the liver. It is mildly laxative. The rhizome-root is the medicinal part.

Use. As a general tonic, gentle aperient. Treatment of all liver ailments, especially jaundice.

Dose. Cut up one rhizome of about six inches in length, into small transverse sections. Steep in wine for twenty-four hours, take a tablespoon three times daily before meals.

Iris Florentina provides the treasured *orris-root* of herbalists and perfume makers. This root gives the sweetly scented orris powder (featured in a recipe in this book).

IVY (*Hedera helix*. Araliaceae). Found as a climber in woodlands, on old walls, cultivated as a house climber. Leaves are heart-shaped. Flowers are small, honey-coloured, very fragrant, sticky. The flowers are beloved by bees and all insects. The dark coloured berries are sought by birds. Both leaves and berries are used. It is a famed fever herb, and a glandular regulator. Used also to expel retained afterbirth.

Use. To calm the blood in all fevers. To reduce dropsical conditions of the body and all enlarged glands, and for mumps: for glandular treatments it is used internally and externally. Externally for inflamed joints, swollen face caused by toothache. Needless to add, it does not cure the dental decay, if present.

Dose. This is a potent herb and should be used in small quantities. Make a Standard brew, using six medium-size leaves to a half-pint of water. Take two tablespoons before meals. For use in removal of retained afterbirth, give two tablespoons every two hours. For external application in other conditions, make a pulp from the leaves or leaves and berries, and apply to the affected area. For stiff joints, make an oil by steeping in salad oil in the recommended way (see Herbal Oils), and massage into the joints. Use this oil also for swollen glands and aching face.

KALE (*Crambe maritima*. Cruciferae). The Kale (marrow-stem and thousand-headed grown largely for farm use) is *Brassica oleracea*, of the Cruciferae family. *Crambe maritima* originally grew wild along the shores of Britain, Western Europe and the Black Sea; under cultivation its blanched sprouts have become a vegetable delicacy. A related plant is the sea radish, *Raphanus maritimus* (Cruciferae), quite a rare species with pungent roots of excellent texture. *Crambe maritima* still found along sea-shores in sandy and stony places, also largely cultivated in gardens. The leaves are rounded and glaucous, flowers are small and white, root is thick and fleshy. A favourite with the Greeks. This plant is exceptionally mineral-rich with much calcium chlorine, phosphorus, potassium and sulphur. A fine blood tonic and nervine. Excellent for the teeth. A remedy for all rheumatic conditions.

Use. As a general tonic for blood and nerves. To improve eyesight and memory. To check decay of teeth and relieve pyorrhoea. For weak blood, unclean blood, rheumatism, sciatica, arthritis, gout, constipation and obesity, also kidney and bladder disorders.

Dose. Eat raw as a salad herb, if possible a few plants daily. Also grind, steep in warm water, flavour with salt and a little red pepper, and drink a cupful of the liquid before meals.

KNAPWEED (*Centaurea nigra*. Compositae). Found in fields and along waysides. Leaves are narrow, small, greyish. Flowers are thistle-form, large and purple and very honey-scented. A fine general tonic. Treatment of glandular disorders. To check haemorrhages. The flowers are used. One of several plants popularly known as 'Bachelor's buttons'.

Use. To restore failing appetite. Treatment of dysentery, gastritis, sour stomach, bad breath. To reduce swollen glands (used internally and externally). Externally as an application for bleeding from nose and mouth, and for anal and vaginal haemorrhages. Here again we must be aware of the danger of concentrating on symptoms rather than causes. As mentioned elsewhere, we must bear in mind that in old times the use of certain herbs was observed to bring about certain effects. Our task today is to discover which properties produce these effects and to deduce therefrom the modern applications. The herb can also be taken internally when the bleeding is severe. Treatment of wounds and running sores.

Dose. Some of the flowers can be eaten raw, especially young ones and buds, cut up in the salad. This is free of prickles and quite edible. Also make a Standard brew of the flowers, for internal and external use. Internally take two tablespoons three times daily. Externally, apply the brew as a cold pack or use as a douche.

LADY'S MANTLE (*Alchemilla vulgaris*. Rosaceae). Found in woodland and shady moist places. Its leaves are cloak-like and pleated, giving this plant its name (it is also a specific for women's ailments). Flowers are numerous, tiny and golden. The true name of this plant is Arabic — *alkemelych*, from the alchemists who were the ancestors' of the chemists, and its name shows the high esteem in which the Arabs held — and still hold — this herb. It is a general tonic for women, for the organs of generation, and if taken from one period to another by barren women will help them to conceive — so the Arabs claim. Also a heart tonic.

Use. Tonic and remedy for the female organs of generation. To cure barrenness and restore normal menstruation. Treatment of heart ailments, also heart tonic. To tone up sluggish blood and fortify weak arteries. Treatment of diabetes and dropsy.

Dose. Some sprigs of the herb eaten raw in salad, twice daily. Or make a Standard brew and drink a small cupful morning and night.

LARKSPUR (*Delphinium consolida*. Ranunculaceae). Found on bank-sides and sandy places. Leaves are dark green and broken. Flowers are intense blue, sometimes greyish. This charming plant is named after the word dolphin, *delphinus*, because of the shape of the upper sepal, considered to resemble that winged animal of the sea. The roots and the seeds are the parts used in herbal medicine. The wild larkspur being an annual, it is not too destructive to take some of the roots after seed dispersal of the plants. Also the whole plant, including the flowers, contains an acid substance which will destroy insect pests. Larkspur was the official remedy for destruction of body lice during the American Civil War. The plant is a remedy for asthma and dropsy.

Use. (External) Treatment against all skin and hair vermin, treatment of asthma (the dry, powdered, plant used as a snuff). Although this plant has also proved to be a remedy for worms and dropsy, I would advise its external use only on account of its potent acid content.

LAUREL (*Laurus nobilis*. Lauraceae). Found wild in Asia Minor, and as a garden shrub, world-wide. Leaves are oval and shiny, frequently gold-speckled. Its flowers are rounded and greenish. Berries dark. The leaves are astringent and therefore of value in dropsical conditions. Laurel leaves are popular in cooking and preserving, enjoyed for their pleasant, bland flavour. Greek peasants use laurel as a chosen flavouring for lentils. They also make a hair tonic from laurel leaves and rosemary.

Use. As a tonic for all the organs of digestion. To promote appetite. Treatment of dropsy, obesity, diabetes, kidney ailments. Externally the leaves are applied to burns and bruises, also soft tumours and all swellings. To flavour soups, olives and cheeses.

Dose. Several leaves taken daily. Soften by holding over hot water. For external use, pulp leaves and also water soften them. Or make a salve with lanolin. As a hair tonic: heat a handful each of laurel leaves and rosemary in a litre of water for half an hour. Do not strain. Rub into hair. Fragrant, strengthening and refreshing.

LAVENDER (*Lavandula spica* and *Lavandula vera*. Labiatae). There are many forms of lavender and all are medicinal and highly valued by the herbalist. Found on dry, sandy land or rocky places. It is much cultivated in gardens, and used in perfumery. Likes coastal areas and mountain-sides. Leaves are thin, narrow, long, greyish; the small flowers are in spikes of blue-purple, they are lipped and very fragrant both when fresh and when dried. As with most strongly scented flowers — especially blue ones — the whole plant is highly nervine. Esteemed as a tea and for flavouring. Externally is used to keep moths from clothing and from dried fruits. Leaves and flowers are used. The latter make an excellent face lotion infused in whey.

Use. As a nerve tonic, treatment of fainting, headache, sunstroke, vomiting, hysteria, paralysis, general weakness of limbs, swelling of limbs. As a mouth wash for those with loose teeth, bad breath. As an asthma inhalation and tea.

Dose. A few of the flower spikes can be eaten raw in the salad. Make a Standard brew of the flowers and take a small cupful morning and night. The flowers can be added to other teas with advantage. To deter moths from clothes closets, place the flowers, spikes and some leaves freely amongst the garments. Or make lavender bags, using open-weave muslin, and fill the bags with the dried flowerets, gathered before midday.

LEMON (*Citrus limonum*. Rutaceae). Found wild in the East. Also found widely in cultivation, likes a sunny climate. Its valued fruits are sold in all parts of the world. Leaves are oval, shiny, fragrant. Flowers are rose-form, white, waxy and very fragrant. Its yellow fruits are too well-known to require description. The lemon tree's leaves and fruit, possess extraordinary healing and general medicinal powers. It is good for almost every ailment, one of the most efficient blood-cleansers and reducers of all fevers. In fever cases there is nothing better to give the patient than diluted lemon juice lightly sweetened with honey. I made this simple remedy the basis of many of my veterinary cures, and it was always very successful.

Use (the fruit). To cleanse the blood, to cool the blood, to expel mucus from all parts of the body. Treatment of all fevers, dysentery, diarrhoea, worm-infestation. Treatment of diabetes, erysipelas. For all skin ailments, pulmonary ailments, jaundice. (The leaves): same uses as the fruit but they are much milder and slower in action. Externally, the raw juice to heal sores, certain abscesses, erysipelas, ringworm. The diluted juice as a lotion for eczema, scalds, burns (one part lemon to three parts water). The very diluted juice, as a lotion for weak or inflamed eyes and for ear ailments (one part lemon to five parts water). The seeds, crushed, are a worm remedy for children. Two teaspoons given on rising, for two weeks.

Dose. In general, half a medium-sized lemon to a cup of water, sweetened with one teaspoon of honey. This cleansing drink is the best means of breaking the night's fast every morning. Similar drink in fever treatments, but using less honey. Those who must, in hot climates, see to the storing of cold water for the day, should add lemon leaves to the water to keep it fresh and give it a pleasant flavour. A few flowers can also be added.

LILY OF THE VALLEY (*Convallaria majalis*. Liliaceae). Found wild in woodlands and damp, shady places. Leaves are oval and grow low from the root; the plant forms a thick mat of underground stems; flowers are waxy white bells, hanging from spikes. It is said to be mildly narcotic. The whole plant is medicinal. The flowers are the most powerful part. The leaves cool inflammations. The roots share also most of the properties of the flowers in a milder form and are gently aperient.

Use. Heart tonic and remedy: not habit-forming. Very calming to the heart, as well as healing. Treatment of nervous ailments, including epilepsy, fits, hysteria. Cures dizziness. Clears the mind and strengthens the memory, soothes nervous irritability. Reduces high blood pressure, reduces risk of apoplexy. For dropsy and all lymph irregularities. Treatment of infestation by thread and round worms: inflamed bowels. Externally the leaves applied to cool all forms of inflammation. From the flowers the French distil their *eau d'or*.

Dose. Two handfuls of the flower spikes in one and a half pints of water, making a Standard brew, or two dessertspoonfuls of the shaved root to same quantity of water. Take a small wineglassful morning and night. A powerful herb, use sparingly.

LINSEED. *See* FLAXSEED.

LIQUORICE (*Glycorrhiza glabra*. Leguminosae). Found wild in many parts of southern Europe on dry stony land. Spain is the principal exporter of stick liquorice. Also largely cultivated as a medicinal and nutritive plant. Leaves are pale green, of many leaflets from a central stalk. Flowers are pale blue and pea-form. Roots are yellow and woody. This herb was much favoured by the great Arabian and medieval herbalists. The root is the part used. It possesses nutritive and laxative properties, and is known to contain female sex hormones. The whole root is used, or the extracted solidified juice which is from crushed, boiled roots obtainable in black sticks. Many sweetmeats are made from liquorice, and they are one of the best confections for satisfying children's desires for such treats. The finely powdered root is an old Arabian remedy for drying up discharging parts of the skin, drying blisters and absorbing all kinds of watery fluids.

Use. Treatment of cough, inflamed throat and for all parts of the pectoral region: pneumonia, pleurisy, tuberculosis. To soothe the stomach and provide a mild laxative for infants and others. Treatment of female infertility, delayed and irregular menstruation. For worms in infants and for chronic constipation. To allay stomach and intestinal cramps. Externally the pulped leaves are softened in hot water and applied to aching ears, externally and inside as ear plugs. The dried, powdered root is used as described above to dry up discharging skin surfaces and blisters. It is also added to flaxseed to make a poultice for treatment of non-malignant tumours.

Babies can be given hard (but not fibrous) pieces of washed liquorice root to chew to help them cut their teeth.

Dose. The solid juice is the most practical way to employ liquorice in medicine. Give approximately three inches of the solid juice sticks daily, dissolved in a half-pint of hot water. Sweeten with honey or brown sugar, take a small wineglass before meals.

LOBELIA (*Lobelia inflata*. Campanulaceae). This is a field plant found mainly in North America where it is commonly called Indian tobacco. Its leaves are pointed and yellowish-green, its flowers hooded and of a brilliant blue (one of its common names being Blue Cardinal flower). Some varieties have red or purple flowers. This is one of the most important herbs of the American Indians, and they have chosen well, for it belongs to a small group of herbs which are virtually cure-alls, being beneficial to the whole body and healing in all ailments. It is especially good for quelling spasms. One species of lobelia, *Lobelia syphilitica* was used by the Canadian Indians in the treatment of all types of veneral diseases. One would hesitate, of course, to claim that this would nowadays and everywhere be the chosen remedy; but nevertheless the well-attested evidence of its effective use over a long period is worth taking into account. It is also useful as an external application for many types of sores, non-malignant ulcers, swellings. The whole plant, including the seed, is used.

Use. In all spasmodic ailments, including heart spasms, convulsions, whooping-cough, chorea and other nervous twitchings, symptoms can be relieved. This herb will relieve vomiting of a spasmodic kind. Lobelia is sometimes called Vomit Weed, and its emetic properties make it valuable in treatment of rabies, when no other help is near. For epilepsy, cramps, obstructions, stomach, liver and bladder disorders. For all fevers, especially typhus, scarlet fever and erysipelas. There are several mid-nineteenth-century references to lobelia's emetic properties, and I have come across a significant note on its use in heavy doses for poisoning unwanted dogs. This is proof enough that lobelia should not be too lavishly used. Externally used as a lotion or ointment for treatment of congested chest, skin ailments.

Dose. A small teaspoon of the crushed leaves, either green or dried. When green use a large teaspoon instead of a small one, pour over this a cupful of hot water (just off the boil), steep and sweeten, and take fasting night and morning. As an emetic, take a half-teaspoon of the dried powdered herbs and pods, add a pinch of cayenne pepper, taken in a cup of warm water. Take the whole dose every half-hour until the stomach is thoroughly cleansed.

As a lotion: steep for one week one ounce of powdered lobelia in a half-pint of apple vinegar, apply to the affected areas, or make a standard brew of lobelia herb and apply as cold compress.

LUCERNE. *See* ALFALFA.

MALLOW (MARSH) (*Althea officinalis*. Malvaceae). The *Malva* (mallow) has a number of species; the *Althea* (marshmallow) is the most interesting. Found in waste places and in gardens. Likes especially salty marshes along sea-shores. Leaves are greyish, softly hairy, toothed, ovate, flowers are mauve, lightly veined with red. The whole plant order of Malvaceae, which includes the *Althaea, Malva* and *Lavatera* genera (the Hollyhock has already been mentioned in this chapter) is one of the most beneficial known to the herbalist, and all the species should be encouraged on farms and in gardens, and never eradicated as useless weeds.

The whole plant is medicinal, from the roots to the fruits.

The leaves when young are a good raw salad herb, and are much eaten by Bedouin Arabs and others. The fruits, called 'cheeses' by peasant children because of their round form, are highly tonic. The roots contain a quantity of mucilaginous matter, also starch, asparagin, albumen (its most valued property), and a crystallizable sugar and a fixed oil. The root in fact contains over half its weight of sweet-tasting mucilage which gives the plant its well-justified reputation, this mucilage having unique healing, soothing and lubricating powers. It is also used in confectionery. The leaves and flowers yield a healing lotion, the roots make a useful poultice, and were once used to check mortification, one ancient name for mallow being 'Mortification Plant'.

The stems of mallow plant are chewed by gypsies, and when the pulp is mixed well with saliva they apply this, warm from the mouth, to inflamed parts of the skin and to sores and swellings. They achieve wonderful cures with this primitive remedy.

Use. Treatment of all lung complaints, also sore throats, hoarseness, sore mouth and gums. All bowel troubles, inflammation, dysentery, diarrhoea, haemorrhage. For irritation of the vagina, internal and external as medicine and as a douche. For breast troubles, soreness, inflammation, swellings. As a lotion to bathe sore or inflamed eyes, and for treatment of styes. Internally and externally for all venereal diseases. Externally, as a lotion or poultice for all skin eruptions, sores, swellings, bruises, sprains.

Dose. A Standard brew of the flowers and leaves. Sweeten with honey and take a wineglass three times daily. Or three or four roots, sliced small and boiled gently for one hour in two pints of water; add honey to sweeten. Take a wineglass three times daily. Use the roots, prepared as above, also externally. The pulped leaves and flowers are applied to the surface of all inflamed areas, or to swellings, wounds, sprains, etc. or used, slightly warmed, as a poultice. Or the leaves crushed, can be steeped in light beer and used as a rub, also for bruises, sprains, etc.

A popular confection known as Marshmallow sweets, is made from the dried, powdered roots. The ingredients are: two ounces marsh-mallow root, and fourteen ounces fine sugar mixed with some mucilage (or gum) tragacanth and water of orange flowers, sufficient to bind all together.

MARIGOLD (*Calendula officinalis*. Compositae). The common or pot marigold is found in cultivated fields, especially in vineyards. Leaves are oval, pale-green, fading rapidly. Flowers are round, many petalled, radiate and of brilliant gold or orange. A 'Herb of the Sun' with much of the sun's power in its flowers, which are the strongest part medicinally, although the whole plant is used. Because marigold flowers are of great benefit to the arteries and veins the Arabs like to feed them to their swift horses — Arab thoroughbred ponies are esteemed the world over.

The mucilage in the flowers and leaves make the plant beneficial for the complexion, and marigolds have long been featured in old-fashioned complexion creams and lotions. As a tea it is both tonic and febrifuge.

108

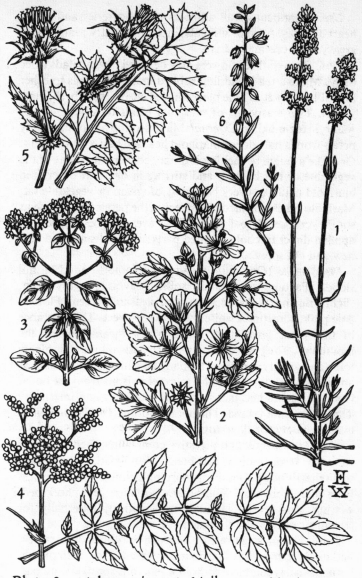

Plate 9.   1. Lavender   2. Mallow   3. Marjoram
4. Meadowsweet 5. Milk Thistle 6. Milkwort

Use. Treatment of all ailments of the arteries and veins; heart diseases. All skin ailments, including spotty complexion, greasy skin, eczema, warts.

Dose. Two or three flowers may be eaten raw in salads twice daily. Make a tea by adding rubbed marigold petals to other herbal teas, such as lime blossom, red clover, speedwell, marjoram. Two teaspoons of marigold petals to a large cup of water, in tea-making. *External:* Make a lotion by boiling gently petals from a half-dozen marigold heads in half a pint of milk. Or make a cream by melting ordinary cold cream or one of the vegetable or nut butters, and stirring in one part of bruised marigold petals to every two parts of cream or vegetable fat. Marigold oil can be made by steeping the petals in oil, such as sunflower (*see* Herbal oils). The leaves can be pulped and applied direct to cool inflamed parts and to cleanse and heal new and old sores.

MARJORAM (*Origanum vulgare*. Labiatae). Found on hill slopes. Favours dry, sandy soils. Leaves are grey-green, slightly downy, highly aromatic and pleasant of scent. Flowers pale pink, sometimes white, very honey-sweet. The fragrance of this plant gives it its name which means 'joy of the mountain'. The plant contains an aromatic oil which is highly tonic and greatly beneficial to man and animals. Much used as an aid to good digestion, and to expel poisons from the body. Good for aches and pains. Is used externally and internally. The whole plant is used. The pot marjoram (*Origanum onites*) is used mainly for flavouring.

Use. Treatment of all digestive complaints, including sour stomach, fermentation, bad breath. Will soothe sore throats and relieve cough. Good for morning sickness, shaky nerves, fears and depression. Will allay nightmares and check bed-wetting. For fevers, jaundice, rheumatism. Externally for treatment of ear- and toothaches, headache, sore throat.

Dose. This pleasant-tasting herb can be rubbed on to salads, and used fresh or dry. The Spanish peasants do not think that lettuce salad is complete without a generous sprinkling of marjoram. Add also to soups and press into white cheese, place some sprigs between brown bread slices. As a tea, a heaped teaspoon of the herb to a half-pint of water.

Externally: a few drops (warmed) of a strong brew of marjoram, strained, put into the ears several times daily, will lessen pains and melt waxy accumulations. For aching teeth drop a few drops of the expressed oil into the cavity or cavities. For sore throat make a strong brew and soak a cotton cloth in this when it is quite hot, and then bind around the throat. Also drink the tea freely, fortified with honey.

MEADOWSWEET (*Filipendula ulmaria*. Rosaceae). Found in damp meadows and along ditch-sides. Leaves are dark green, shiny, somewhat like rose leaves, but thornless. Flowers are in creamy plumes and most sweetly scented. As with lavender, place bunches or sachets of the flowers in linen closets and wardrobes. The plant is a proved fever herb, of use in dysentery, and will improve the complexion. The flowers are used.

Use. Treatment of all fevers, blood disorders, high blood-pressure, diabetes. For dysentery, diarrhoea, colic. Externally as a complexion tonic.

Dose. A handful of the flowers made into a Standard brew. Take a wineglass of it, sweetened with honey, morning and night. Externally: make a lotion by steeping flower heads in shallow dishes of water (preferably rain-water) placed in the sun. This is an old Somerset gypsy treatment: dew collected from teasel and other plants is also added to improve the lotion.

MIGNONETTE (*Reseda lutea*. Resedaceae). Found in shady places, waste places. Also cultivated in gardens, especially the fragrant mignonette, *Reseda odorata*. Leaves are small, silvery, flowers are in spikes, minute, inconspicuous, of brownish yellow, sweetly scented. The name *Reseda* means 'calm', and indicates the narcotic properties of this plant. Provence peasants would stuff pillows with *Reseda odorata* in the same way as English country folk would stuff pillows with hops, to induce sweet sleep. The plant has other medicinal properties; soothing irritated nerve ends, and as a wound herb, especially when added to other wound herbs to enhance the pain-relieving properties.

Use. To calm the nerves, used both internally and externally. Treatment of asthma, hay-fever.

Dose. Make a Standard brew and take two tablespoons three times daily. Or the Standard brew can be used externally as a wound lotion and to soothe inflamed eyes. External. Stuff muslin pillows with *Reseda odorata*, as a remedy against sleeplessness and nightmares.

MILK THISTLE (*Cardus* (*Silybum*) *Marianus*. Compositae). Found on waste land and in pastures. Likes rich organic soil. Leaves are grey with veins of silver-white, large, with prickly edges. Flowers are large, thistle-form purple, and the involucre prickly and barbed. The name of the flower *marianum* — is sometimes explained thus: a drop of milk from the breast of the Virgin Mary is said to have fallen on this thistle as she was cutting thistle fodder to feed her donkey. The thistle then became medicinal and edible. The word *Cardus* shows that the species were once used for carding wool. The word comes from the Celtic and Gaelic word for a card for combing wool. The leaves of this thistle are a wonderful remedy for healing wounds and sores. The young shoots can be eaten in salads. The seeds are used in rabies and epilepsy. A species grows in the Holy Land, also called after the Virgin Mary, *Silybum marianum* (see p. 91). This is also a milky-veined thistle. On good ground it can reach man-height. The young shoots, called in Arabic *Khurfesh*, are gathered and eaten by the Bedouin shepherds and other Arabs. I have eaten quantities when living in or visiting Bedouin tents: this is a very refreshing salad food. The green fleshy stems are the best part.

Use. A wound herb. Also as a medicinal salad, blood-cleansing, a jaundice remedy, treatment of anaemia, rickets, scurvy, *petsas* — those big, deep sores found in eastern Mediterranean countries. Externally for wounds, sores. The seeds to cure fits, epilepsy, once used against rabies.

Dose. The hearts of several plants eaten daily as a salad herb. Collect before the thistles become tough and spiky: trim off any soft prickles. Externally, the young, large leaves are trimmed of their prickles, with scissors, and gently crushed, then bound over wounds and sores. They will turn black later from the heat and foul matter drawn from sores, *petsas*, etc. Eat a dessertspoonful of the seeds, morning and night, in treatment of those ailments for which they are intended.

MILKWORT (*Polygala vulgaris*. Polygalaceae). Found on heaths and other sandy places. A tiny plant reaching only several inches. Leaves are tiny, narrow. Flowers are flat and bright blue. This little plant has long been valued for increasing milk yield, and is therefore indicated for nursing mothers and milch animals. Named from the Greek, *gala*, milk, its name translates as 'much milk'.

Use. To increase flow of breast milk. To cool the blood.

Dose. A handful eaten raw twice daily.

MINT (*Mentha viridis*. Labiatae). Found in moist places, also amongst rocks. Widely cultivated (*Mentha spicata* and *M. rotundifolia*) in gardens for culinary use. Leaves are narrow, rough, very fragrant, possessing the peculiar mint scent and flavour. Flowers are thin spikes of pale mauve, and are also highly scented with mint odour. A wild water-mint grows along ditch sides. It was once esteemed as a cure for frigidity in both sexes, and even today is used as a tonic for bulls and stallions when their sexual powers are waning. The Arabs drink mint tea frequently, to ensure virility, also as a social drink, because Moslems are not wine drinkers. The only negative quality of this excellent herb is that it is apt to diminish milk secretion, and therefore should not be taken by nursing mothers.

Mint soothes as well as excites, quells stomach pains and gas, and has an altogether beneficial effect on the stomach and digestive tract. Will restore failing appetite and allay rheumatic pains.

Use. Treatment of infertility and lack of normal sexual desire. To cure disorders of the digestive system, including acid stomach, flatulence, gastritis, diarrhoea, dysentery. As a headache remedy, taken as a tea and applied externally as a cold pack to the forehead. A stronger treatment for headache is to steep slices of raw potato in a cold, strong brew of mint, and apply the potato slices to the head, placing a cloth wrung out in the water, over them to keep them in place. Change the potato slices at intervals. To treat suppression of urine, also suppressed menstruation. To quell vomiting and general nausea. Externally as a rub for rheumatism and arthritis and stiff joints.

Dose. To be eaten in salads, a few sprigs daily. Or make a strong tea sweetened with honey. Take a cupful after meals. Externally: crush, heat gently for a few minutes. Then steep in apple vinegar overnight, apply as a rub. For headache, use the mint vinegar lotion cold. Steep a cotton cloth in this and lay this across the forehead. Renew frequently: an *excellent* headache remedy.

MISTLETOE (*Viscum album*. Loranthaceae). Found in woodlands and orchards, growing as a parasite, lodged in bark crevices of the host treee. The seeds are often planted by the mistle-thrush. Leaves are horseshoe shape and yellowish. The flowers are inconspicuous, greenish, and produce round, white, rather glutinous berries. This is a plant of legend because of its effect upon the nerves, soothing and calming. For that reason, in ancient herbal books mistletoe was often called the 'Golden Bough'. It is described as a remedy for epilepsy.

Use. Treatment of epilepsy, St. Vitus's Dance. Also for hysteria, convulsions, delirium, weak nerves, and to calm over-excited heart. Externally as a rub for stiff joints, swellings, and to soothe burning piles.

Dose. Three or four berries taken fasting, night and morning, or can be macerated in a teaspoon of honey. (Not recommended for infants.) Externally: merely pound up a handful of berries and apply as a rub.

MULLEIN (*Verbascum thapsus*. Scrophulariaceae). Found along waysides and on neglected land. Leaves are broad, grey and very downy, giving the plant one of its common names — 'Blanket Herb'. The flowers are in tall spikes and are of yellow, rose-form. This is a famed old household remedy and

HERBAL MATERIA MEDICA

a favourite of the American Indians. It is valued for its effect
on the chest area, and for that reason has always been a stand-
by remedy for lung ailments in cattle, another of its common
names being 'Cow Lungwort'. It is equally good for humans
in this respect. The leaves and flowers are used. The flowers
must be stored in tin containers for they turn black in bright
light, once off the plant. Yet another name is 'candle light'
the down being used as wicks.

Use. Treatment of cough, pneumonia, pleurisy, bronchitis,
tuberculosis, asthma (for asthma internally and as an
inhalant). Also a remedy for bleeding from the mouth, nose,
lungs, bowels. Treatment of dropsy, all bowel complaints, and
hay-fever. In treatment of dysentery, and bleeding from the
bowels, boil in new milk some mullein leaves, a dessertspoon to
half a pint of milk, add honey, nutmeg, cinnamon, and take
two tablespoons of this drink after each bowel movement, or at
least three times daily. For external use make hot fomentations
from a cloth wrung out in a brew of the leaves or flowers, and
apply to swollen glands, stiff neck, mumps, and to the throat
for inflamed tonsils. Some vinegar can be added to the fomentation with advantage.

A tea of the flowers will promote sleep and soothe headaches. Use this tea too as an application for warts.

Dose. Make a Standard brew of the leaves and/or flowers.
Take a small cupful night and morning. Or steep the leaves in
milk (see above, under *Use*).

Externally, as fomentation (also see above). For asthma, use
an old kettle, place within a heaped tablespoonful of the
leaves, cut fine, pour on to this some boiling water, and inhale
the steam through the spout (keeping the head beneath a
towel). This same inhalation can be used for hay-fever,
congestion of the nose, and all sinus troubles.

MUSTARD ((Black) *Brassica nigra* (White) *Sinapis alba*.
Cruciferae). Found on waste land and in gardens. Also
cultivated as a pasture herb. Leaves are cress-form, hot, biting.
Flowers are intense yellow, cross-form, also hot and biting.
Seeds are long, narrow, also very hot. The herb is an important

115

antiseptic tonic. It is used both in medicine and to cleanse pastures. As a green manure crop, mustards are dug in just at flowering time. Mustard is also a poultice and plaster herb. In external application it acts as an irritant and excitant: in this form it is valuable in treatment of paralysis and pectoral complaints. The condiment is usually prepared from the seeds of Black Mustard.

Use. Treatment of poor appetite, flatulence, bad breath. Treatment of colds, catarrh, pneumonia. Externally as a poultice or rubbing remedy, to relieve internal and external inflammations, congested lungs, paralysed limbs, rheumatic and arthritic pains and stiffness.

Dose. Eat the young leaves freely as a salad herb. A handful can be eaten easily, daily, as a spring tonic and general blood remedy. When a cold is threatening chew a teaspoon of the seeds several times during the day to expel the accumulating mucus. To make a mustard poultice, use a handful of mustard flour (obtainable from grocers and pharmacies) to a handful of bran, make a paste with hot water: apply hot. To make a mustard plaster, to every handful of ground mustard add three parts of wholewheat flour. Mix into a pliable paste with hot water. Then add further some hot vinegar (about two teaspoons of vinegar to a half-pint measure of the mustard-wholewheat flour mixture). Spread on a piece of cloth and apply hot over the area to be treated: chest, kidneys, paralysed areas. In cases of sensitive skin where blisters may be provoked, add the white of an egg to every half-pint measure of the mixture. Mustard baths are a de-congestant.

NASTURTIUM (*Tropaeolum*. Cruciferae). Found wild as an escape from gardens. Well known as a garden plant, creeping and climbing. Leaves are umbrella shape, frail, brilliant green, conspicuously veined. Flowers of brilliant colours, especially oranges and reds, spurred, single or double. The whole plant has a hot, biting character, especially the seeds which were once much used as a caper-like pickle. The plant is an important antiseptic herb, also vermifuge (especially the seeds).

116

Use. As an antiseptic for the blood and digestive organs; to stimulate appetite. To cure nervous depression, tiredness, poor sight. Treatment of all worms. An excellent remedy for digestive gripings is a teaspoon of the seeds ground into a powder and given in enough cold water to liquefy, every three hours. As a table pickle the fruits are a substitute for capers, whole in apple vinegar, spiced with cloves, laurel leaves and thyme. Externally: A poultice of the seeds crushed and placed on flannel wrung out in hot water, for application to abscesses, boils, styes and old sores.

Dose. Three or four leaves eaten raw in the salad; raw flowers can also be used. For worms treatment, eat six to ten seeds, best when eaten green. Eat these seeds fasting, night and morning.

NETTLE (*Urtica dioica.* Urticaceae). Found over waste land and in hedgerows. The leaves are serrated, dull green, hairy. These leaves possess an acrid fluid (formic acid) which burns the human skin, causing small blisters — hence the common name of this plant — Stinging Nettle. Flowers are green-yellow, in clusters, small. The Roman pill nettle species has large seed capsules like green balls and was planted extensively by Romans as a rheumatic remedy, for flogging the human skin to increase the blood flow. Also, as with bee and ant stings, the formic acid was considered beneficial. To this day bruised leaves of stinging nettles are rubbed on the skin in treatment of chronic rheumatism. The whole plant is powerfully medicinal, from the roots to the seed.

Use. The root: treatment of dropsy, lymphatic ailments, to expel gravel and stones from any organ in which they have formed, especially from the kidneys. The leaves: as a vegetable (lightly boiled, for several minutes only until softened and the stinging quality is neutralized, then add some flaked oats and good butter); to cleanse the blood, tone up the whole system; as cure for anaemia, rheumatism, sciatica, arthritis, obesity, infertility. A Standard brew made from the leaves, to expel excess mucus from all parts of the body. Externally, use as a hair wash — a rinse and scalp massage. Will improve the

117

colour and texture of the hair and remove dandruff. As a nerve and tissue excitant, in treatment of chronic rheumatism, paralysis, stiffness of joints, failing muscular strength. The gypsy method is to bind fresh-cut plants into a bunch and beat the affected parts with this until great heat is created in the limb. Then cotton cloths, soaked in cold vinegar, are applied and after several hours the nettle flogging is repeated. Many cures of chronic cases have been achieved with this primitive treatment — and, as already written, the Romans planted nettles especially for this curative purpose. The leaves, applied fresh to bleeding wounds, will often act effectively within a few minutes.

Flowers and seed (the nettle produces much seed): as a hair rinse and for scalp massage. Heated gently in wine and swallowed as a cure for diarrhoea and dysentery. Made into a Standard brew, serves as a blood-cleanser and to expel worms.

Dose. Eat the boiled leaves as a vegetable as freely as you would eat spinach or other greens. No other green vegetable excels the nettle in mineral and vitamin content. This is one of the world's most chlorophyll-rich plants. Standard brew of the leaves: a wine-glass three times daily. Nettle juice can be made in a juicer.

Standard brew of the flowers and/or seed: Similar dose to the leaves. A lotion for aching feet: brew one handful of nettle leaves, and one of marsh-mallow leaves, in three-quarters of a pint of whey or plain water. Use warm.

NETTLE (White or Blind. *Lamium album*. Labiatae). Known commonly also as Stingless Nettle or Dead Nettle, is not related to the Common Nettle. Found in woodlands and as a garden weed. Leaves are nettle-form, downy. Flowers are hooded, white, two-lipped, in whorls. Entirely stingless.

Use. To stem bleeding, especially nasal bleeding, bleeding from uterus, bowels, over-heavy menses. As a douche and as local application (on cloths soaked in a Standard brew).

OATS (*Avena sativa*. Gramineae). Found in corn-fields and on banksides and under cultivation in pastures. Leaves are typical grass-form, darkish, brittle, spikelets are drooping and frail, the grains are awned and turn dark gold when ripe. Oats are a strength-giving cereal. Low in starch, high in mineral content (especially potassium and phosphorus, also magnesium and calcium). Particularly rich in vitamin B, with some of the rare E and G also. Highly nerve-tonic and bone-building, also used externally as a skin tonic (the finely ground meal). A basic food of the hardy Scottish Highlanders.

Use. As a nutritive food, nerve tonic, blood tonic, hair tonic. Remedy for rickets. Important for ensuring strong nails and teeth.

Dose. Oats cannot be eaten raw, unless taken as flakes, when the slight heat used during their flaking dispenses with the need to cook them further and they can be eaten dry, raw, or with milk poured over.

Externally, fine oatmeal makes an excellent poultice, and is applied to the skin as a cleansing rub. Also the meal, placed in cotton bags, is rubbed over the skin as a complexion treatment, some drops of perfume being added. The bags are squeezed out in warm water and a milky lotion is produced.

OPIUM POPPY (*Papaver somniferum*. Papaveraceae). Found on hillsides and waste land. Also widely cultivated. Leaves are grey-green, juicy. Flowers are of typical poppy form, white or white purple shaded, with a bitter scent. The seed capsules and seeds are the most important medicinal part. The virtues of opium have been known to mankind since most ancient times. It is one of the few herbs widely used by the orthodox medical profession which, so far, has no synthetic rival. The opium poppy yields a milky juice highly esteemed for its narcotic and stimulating properties. This juice contains many active principles, the most valued being morphine and codeia.

The white juice is collected from the unripe seed capsules, slits being made all around them, and the exuding milky juice is then carefully collected. This is allowed to solidify into cakes, baked in the sun until of a deep brown colour. The cakes are then coated with dried poppy leaves and seed and can be stored without losing their medicinal powers. The natural juice is harmless, a gentle soother of all organs of the body and lightly tonic. The prepared drug is poisonous and should be used with great care. Properly used it is beneficial to allay pain (especially in cancer and other painful disorders): misused, it can destroy the human brain and body. One of the worst effects of the prepared drug is its influence on the intestinal nerves. It over-soothes them and causes them to become torpid, thus bringing on incurable constipation, so that opium addicts turn into white-fleshed beings with fetid breath. I saved the life of my daughter when she was a few months old, and given up by Spanish doctors: I made a brew of opium poppy heads, and fed teaspoonfuls of this to her day and night for several days. But this is a drastic remedy, not to be carried out by beginners in herbal medicine.

Use. To relieve pain, soothe the nerves, give gentle sleep. Treatment of aching teeth, eyes, ears.

Dose (The seed capsules). Make a Standard brew and give a tablespoon three times daily before meals, sweetened with honey. Externally, use the Standard brew as a vaginal or anal douche in treatment of irritation of vagina or bowels, and for inflammation generally. Squeeze juice from the capsules or from the base of the capsules after picking, dilute with two parts of warm water, and apply to cavities of aching teeth or drop into the ears. For inflamed or burning eyes, bathe with a Standard brew of the dried capsules.

ORCHIS (Early purple) (*Orchis maculata*. Orchidaceae). Found in meadows and pastures. Likes damp ground. Leaves are long, shiny, with dark spots. Flowers in spikes, rose-purple. Flowers are of peculiar orchid-form and very beautiful. The root tubers are the most important part of this herb, and give it the Arabic name of *Sahleb* — and the Turkish — *Salep*. These tubers yield a flour which is widely used in the East as food and medicine. (See p. 195). The tubers are dug up after the plant has flowered, are then carefully sun-dried, crushed and eaten raw. Or they are made into a flour, by grinding the sun-ripened tubers, mixing with honey, and hot water is stirred in slowly until the desired strength is reached. Then the

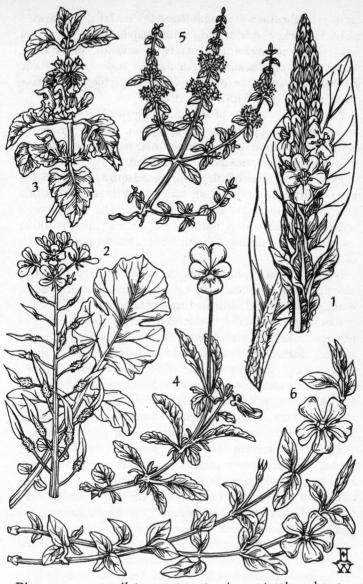

Plate 10.   1. Mullein   2. Mustard   3. Nettle (white)
4. Pansy   5. Pennyroyal   6. Periwinkle

drink is further thickened with the addition of slightly warmed milk. In Turkey, Arabia and Persia, salep is highly prized as a beverage for the weaning of infants, for invalids, for the aged, and for restoring sexual vigour to men and women whose powers are waning, or for those who are infertile. Also to give strength to women with birth problems.

Use. For the weaning of infants. As a general restorative. As an aphrodisiac. Treatment of exhaustion, general weakness, infertility, abortion, poor appetite, anaemia. For weak nerves, twitching of limbs, trembling, nightmares.

Dose. Two ounces of salep flour mixed into a thin paste with three-quarters of a pint of hot water, then three-quarters of a pint of warm milk are added, and honey. Can be flavoured with ground cinnamon, nutmeg, etc. Take a cupful morning and night. Give during difficult labour, but without addition of milk.

NOTE   Orchids of all kinds are now a protected plant in most countries, so the salep orchid should be cultivated at home if culinary and medicinal use is to continue.

PANSY (*Viola tricolor.* Violaceae). Found on heaths and moors. Leaves are small, scanty. Flowers bright purple, viola-shaped, marked with yellow and a little white. Popular name 'Heart's-ease', famed for its beneficial effects upon the heart, both as tonic and remedy. Known to aid speed for athletes.

Use. Treatment of heart weakness, pains and ailments. High blood-pressure. Skin ailments, breast swellings, boils, abscesses.

Dose. A tablespoon of the herb eaten raw, early morning, fasting. For heart pains, make a Standard brew, sweeten with honey, and drink a wineglass every four hours.

PARSLEY (*Petroselinum sativum.* Umbelliferae). Found on dry rocky soil and cultivated in gardens. Leaves are curled or plain and of an intense green colour. They have a characteristic odour and flavour, due to a substance called Apiol. Considered useful in cancer prevention and treatment; and taken when cancer is prevalent in families. Parsley is beneficial to the urinary system, and is used for bladder and kidney complaints. The root is a safe and effective aperient. All parts of the plant are used including the seed. Only the Spanish peasants warn against eating too much parsley; they say it will make people look older than their true years!

Use. Disorders of bladder and kidneys, gravel, stone, congestion, cystitis, dropsy, jaundice, rheumatism, arthritis, sciatica. Also anaemia, rickets. Treatment of female ailments. The bruised leaves steeped in vinegar will relieve swollen breasts. The cold leaves, bruised and worn inside a bodice around the breasts, will help to dry up the milk when the weaning of infants is desired.

Dose. A handful of fresh parsley eaten once or twice daily in salad. Or it can be chopped fine and put into sandwiches, or mixed with white cottage cheese. A strong tea of the leaves provides a good drink for diabetics. Make a tea from the seeds, using a tablespoon of seed to one pint of water. Bring to the boil, steep until cold, and then drink a cupful morning and night. This same tea, when steeped at least seven hours and rubbed into the hair, will clear away head lice. A hot lotion of the seeds and/or leaves will soothe all kinds of insect stings. Massage the head scalp with the same seeds/leaves lotion to stimulate growth of hair, check baldness and remove dandruff. Some parsley should be cultivated in pots, for winter use.

PARSNIP (Wild) (*Pastinaca sativa*. Umbelliferae). Found in field borders and in pastures; the parsnip cultivated in gardens and fields is *Peucedanum sativum*. Leaves are serrated, rough, generally shining due to the potassium content of this plant; downy below. Flowers inconspicuous, yellowish, roots tapering with stringy ends, white inside, strongly scented. Parsnip is highly medicinal, tonic, bland, and makes a good drawing poultice.

Use. Nutritive, tonic. Can be eaten by diabetics, being highly rich in minerals and medicinal and quite low in sugar content. Treatment of all urinary ailments, including stone, gravel. Treatment of dropsy, as a poultice. Pulp up the root raw, and apply direct to the affected place. Will relieve abscesses, boils and swellings.

Dose. Use plentifully as a vegetable, grated, raw. If lightly steamed, and served with white sauce, seasoned with parsley, you have a typical French peasant dish.

PENNYROYAL (*Mentha pulegium.* Labiatae). Found alongside brooks and streams and in marshy meadows. A diminutive plant. Leaves are tiny, stalkless, pointed, flowers are tiny, of lilac colour, and in clusters. The name *pulegium* is from the Latin for 'flea', and denotes the power of this plant as an insecticide. It is also a powerful mosquito repellent and is much used for this purpose by the Arabs, the leaves and flowers being well pulped and then rubbed on to the skin. It is used also for bites from snakes and dogs. A good remedy for female ills. The distilled oil of pennyroyal possesses soothing and warming powers and is used to promote perspiration and to expel phlegm: helpful in all pulmonary ailments.

Use. Treatment of catarrh, cough, pneumonia, bronchitis, pleurisy and tuberculosis. Most female complaints, especially irregular or suppressed menstruation (should be taken hot at night-time following a hot bath). For uterine ulcers, exhaustion after child-birth. Should not be taken by pregnant women. Treatment of headache, toothache, earache, as a mouth wash and throat gargle. For digestive ailments, including stomach gas, sour stomach, failing appetite. Externally for skin ailments, for bites of all kinds, to repel fleas, ticks, mosquitoes.

Dose. A Standard brew. Take two tablespoons before meals, three times daily. For external use, steep the herb in vinegar and apply, or make a herbal oil infusion (see Herbal Oils); as mosquito repellent, rub the fresh herb on to the skin where exposed to insects.

PEONY (*Paeonia officinalis.* Ranunculaceae). Found on hillsides and in pastures: also cultivated in gardens, for its beautiful red or white heavily scented flowers. Leaves are wide, winged, stems thick and reddish, flowers solitary, large, round of form, richly coloured, heavily perfumed. Evidence that this plant has valuable medicinal properties is found in its name, derived from Paeon, the great herbalist of the ancient Greeks, mentioned by Theophrastus. The root is the chief medicinal part, and is narcotic and anti-spasmodic. It is especially valued for treatment of epilepsy. The flowers are male and female and yield a syrupy extract. The wild peony is more powerfully medicinal than the garden variety but lacks perfume.

Use. Treatment of all nervous disorders, especially those of a spasmodic nature, chorea, epilepsy, twitchings — including twitchings of eyelids. Also for rheumatism, dropsy, glandular ailments.

Dose. Make a brew from the roots. Flake the roots finely and place one ounce in three-quarters of a pint of cold water. Bring to the boil, simmer gently for fifteen minutes (keeping covered throughout). Remove from the fire and steep for three hours. Then strain and add a teaspoon of brandy or rum to every small wineglass of the brew. Take two tablespoons of the mixture before meals.

In rheumatism and glandular ailments take internally, also rub the affected parts with the brew, not forgetting the addition of brandy or rum.

PEPPERMINT (*Mentha piperita*. Labiatae). Found in damp meadows and verges of woodland, also widely cultivated in gardens. Leaves are downy, greyish, flowers are pale purple, in whorls, and very aromatic. The plant yields a warming oil. Indeed, few plants excel peppermint for its warming, heartening qualities, and it makes a far more effective nerve-stimulating drink than either coffee or common (Indian or China) tea, without sharing their harmful properties. This herb cleanses and strengthens the entire body. Good to take after shock, or swimming cramps, and for a feeling of faintness.

Use. A general tonic for the whole body, especially for the digestive and nervous system. Take many hot cups as a headache remedy, in preference to aspirin or similar pain-relief drugs.

For gas in stomach, stomach pains, cramps, indigestion, nausea. For constipation, painful menstruation. To banish mental depression, induce sleep, cure fainting attacks.

Dose. A cupful of a Standard brew, taken morning and night, or after meals in digestive troubles. Take more frequently — as desired — for headache treatment, and before bedtime for sleeplessness. Sweeten with honey.

PERIWINKLE (*Vinca major* and *Vinca minor*. Apocynaceae). Found in woodlands and on shady banksides. A trailing plant. Leaves are dark green, glossy, oval and evergreen. Flowers are starry, pale-blue with lighter centres. It is an important nerve herb and a powerful astringent. Used to control an over-abundant flow of breast milk, and to dry off the milk supply during weaning of infants. Externally used as an astringent.

Use. Treatment of nervous ailments, including nervous debility. To check haemorrhages, internal and external, including bleeding from nose, vagina, deep wounds. To allay prolonged chronic diarrhoea. To control excess of milk and dry up dripping teats (internal and external treatment). To dry up deep wounds, sores, ulcers.

Dose. A Standard brew. Take two tablespoons, with honey, morning and night. Externally, apply the same brew, cold, without the honey.

PIMPERNEL (Scarlet) (*Anagallis arvensis*. Primulaceae). Found on waste land and in fields. A tiny plant, almost thread-like. Leaves simple, tiny, yellowish green. Flowers solitary, rounded, open only in sunlight, and are of an intense red. The medicinal properties of this plant are more important than its appearance suggests. It is an ancient peasant remedy for the bites of snakes, scorpions and rabid animals, and was used both internally and externally for this purpose. Will calm rages in adults and children, if they can be induced to drink it. There is also a blue pimpernel.

Use. Treatment of stings, bites. To soothe nettle rash, poison ivy rash; treatment of jaundice, dropsy, swellings. Though milder, the blue is similarly used; excellent for hepatitis.

Dose. Macerate the whole plant and steep in cold water in sunlight for several hours a handful of herb to a small cup of water. Take a tablespoon three times daily. Make a Standard brew for external use (also when there is no sunlight available). Take a tablespoon three times daily. For bites, etc. crush the whole herb and apply direct to the place affected.

PLANTAIN (*Plantago major*. Plantaginacaea). Found on waste land and in fields. But will grow anywhere, even in the middle of pathways. Its leaves are in flat rosettes, and are oval or lanceolate and prominently veined. The flowering spike is peculiar and has a look of a slender bulrush in its narrow form and brownish flowers massed together into a narrow spike. This is a major wound herb and is also valuable in many ailments where internal inflammation has developed.

The name of this herb is derived from *planta*, foot, owing to the flat form of the leaves. The leaves and root yield a soothing and healing mucilage which is somewhat like linseed, but even more powerfully medicinal. Plantain is an old-fashioned herb and a favourite of the American Indians and the gypsies everywhere. The latter used to do a profitable trade in peddling plantain ointment as a general cure-all. Used internally and externally it was once a treatment for syphilis. It has a great reputation for treatment of the urinary organs, and for checking excessive discharges from the body, whether from bowels or from uterus. The young leaves, sliced, can be eaten as a salad herb.

Gives speedy relief when applied to all kinds of bites and stings, and has been used against all kinds of bites, ranging from dogs' to ants'. Excellent for all skin ailments, the crushed leaves being applied direct. Plantain is also used very successfully as a poultice herb.

Use. For dysentery, diarrhoea, ulcers, fevers. Externally, for wounds, sores, ulcers, skin rashes, eczema, erysipelas, boils and abscesses, scalds and burns. Also for first aid for all kinds of bites and stings, including those of snakes, scorpions, poisonous spiders. For application to piles, aching teeth, inflamed eyes (using the root or leaves).

Dose. Eat a few young leaves raw in the daily salad. Or make a Standard brew of the leaves, finely cut, or from the sliced root; the root requires boiling for approximately five minutes and then steeping for several hours. Take a wineglass of the brew of either leaves or root, morning and night. An ointment can be made by pounding up the leaves and mixing into melted cold cream or into melted vegetable fats. As a poultice apply either the pulped leaves or crushed and boiled roots, hot, on pieces of linen, and bind into place.

POPPY (Red, Field) (*Papaver Rhoeas*. Papaveraceae). Found in corn-fields, waste places, gardens. Leaves are fern-like, hairy, silvery green. Flowers are of typical poppy-form, of an intense red, the petals often having a blue-black base. The heads droop when in bud, petals are shed very readily.

This plant is valued as a gentle narcotic. All parts except the root are medicinal. The leaves are used as a tonic tea, the petals for the throat and pectoral area, also in fevers. The seed capsules are the part with special pain-relieving qualities, and the seeds are considered highly tonic and are used in food as well as in medicine.

Use. The leaves and flowers — especially the flowers, for catarrh, cough, inflamed throat and lungs, pneumonia, pleurisy. To promote sweating in fevers and in lung ailments and to soothe the patient. For relief of asthma and hay fever.

The seed capsules as a nervine, to soothe over-excitability of the mind and body, to induce mild sleep. Externally as an eye lotion, especially for smarting, inflammation, ulcers, pink-eye. Treatment of earache, local twitchings. The seed as a tonic food and for flavouring and garnishing; for sprinkling on bread. Turkish peasants make tonic cakes from roasted poppy seed mixed with olive oil, honey and roasted flour to bind the mixture. In Israel, poppy-seed cake is sold in most cake shops.

Dose. The whole plant, leaves to flowers, made into a Standard brew. Take two tablespoons morning and night. As a gentle narcotic, make a strong tea from six of the seed capsules to a half-pint of water, prepare by Standard method, take a cupful three or four times during the day, every two hours when relief of pain is the object. Use the seed-capsules lotion for treatment of local aches and inflammations of eyes, ears, and for headaches.

As a tonic, take a dessertspoon of the seeds every morning, preferably raw, unroasted. Wash through a small-mesh strainer before taking, to remove the dust which is usually

128

present in poppy seed. The white juice from the base of unripe seed capsules can be applied as a wart remover.

PRIMROSE (*Primula vulgaris*. Primulaceae). Found in woodlands, on bank-sides and by streams. Leaves are oval, crinkled, green-yellow. Flowers are solitary, frail, pale yellow, starry, sweetly scented. Another gypsy favourite, especially of the English gypsies. All parts of the plant are used. It is efficacious in removing excess acid from the system.

Use. Treatment of over-acidity, also high blood-pressure, rheumatism, arthritis, sciatica. Also for fits, paralysis, gall-stones, worms. The seed heads when fully ripe are a good emetic.

Dose. One handful of the flowers once daily, eaten raw (may be shredded up and mixed with honey to render them more palatable). Three or four leaves can be eaten raw as salad.

PUFFBALL (Fungi). When crushed and applied to wounds will check excessive bleeding and promote healing. Learnt from the Manouche gypsies of Alsace-Lorraine.

PUMPKIN (*Cucurbita maxima*. Cucurbitaceae). Cultivated in gardens. Leaves are vine-shaped, rough. Flowers tubular, brilliant orange, fall early. Flowers, fruit and seeds are all medicinal. Magic properties have since ancient times been associated with pumpkin seed. The flowers make a tonic tea and stuffed with rice provide a food. The fruit is nutritive, minerals- and vitamin-rich, tonic, soothing. The seeds are nervine, tonic, and also have remarkable powers for expelling tape-worm. (In the Doctrine of Signatures — which is a belief that the form of plants, their roots, leaves, flowers, fruits, seeds, resemble the organ or ailment for which they are curative — the seeds of pumpkin resemble the flat white segments of the tape-worm.) The bruised leaves repel flies.

Use. The flower as a reviving tea. The fruit (vegetable) as a tonic food, to strengthen the blood, as an anaemia and rickets remedy. Also soothes delicate stomachs. Externally, slices of roasted pumpkin, cut from the outer skin, make a good drawing poultice for the treatment of boils and abscesses. Should be applied as hot as can be tolerated. The seeds are used against tape-worm. In acetone, they kill mosquito larvae.

Dose. Of the flowers make a Standard brew for use as a tea. Three of the flowers to a half-pint of water. Of the fruit, several large slices eaten daily. It is not very palatable, but if possible take a portion of the pumpkin raw, grated finely. The rest can be lightly boiled or roasted.

Tape-worm treatment with pumpkin seed

Use sun-dried or oven-dried seeds. Use skimmed, raw milk as the medium for the mixture made up as follows. Two tablespoons of well-crushed, dried pumpkin seed. One tablespoonful unrefined castor oil, one tablespoonful honey.

Having fasted the previous day on fruit juices only, drink the pumpkin seed mixture the following early morning on an empty stomach. After 1½ hours drink a purging mixture made from one tablespoonful castor oil, one tablespoon honey, stirred into half a cup of lemon juice, made from the juice of three lemons diluted with several tablespoonfuls of tepid water.

The patient should remain in bed until the purge has worked. And for the rest of the day and the following day, remain on a light diet of skimmed, diluted milk and flaked oats. No cure is obtained unless the *head* of the worm is expelled.

Raw pumpkin seeds, well chewed, may be taken daily to prevent worm infestation. Similarly, seeds of all varieties of melon, of cucumber and of papaya may be chewed and swallowed as a vermifuge. Arabian camel drivers chew watermelon seeds to increase endurance and hold thirst at bay on long journeys.

All these seeds may be lightly sprinkled with salt and water and gently roasted for storing in jars or tins and taking as an occasional tonic.

PURSLANE (*Portulaca oleracea*. Portulaceae). Found in damp pastures and in orchards or on dry land after heavy rains. Leaves are vivid green, small, opposite, fleshy. Stems also fleshy. Flowers, small, bright yellow, forming many small black seeds.

Although this is a common weed in most parts of the world, I had never used it or heard about it until I lived in coconut

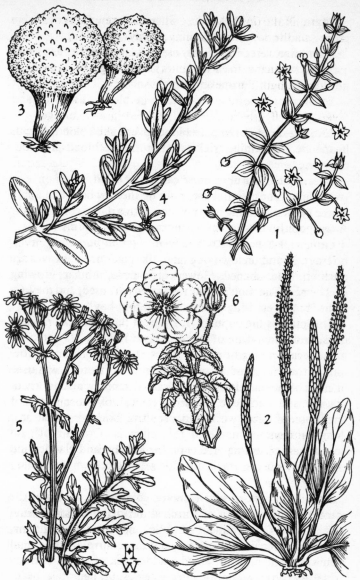

Plate II.   1. Pimpernel   2. Plantain   3. Puffball
            4. Purslane   5. Ragwort   6. Rock Rose

plantations of tropical Mexico, where it was our only available green salad food, always cooling, always refreshing.

I have discovered its popular use in Arab countries as a salad food and medicine. In earlier times it was cultivated as a valued pot-herb in both Europe and North America. The whole plant is refrigerant, soothing, excellent in blood disorders and fevers. It is slightly laxative and the seeds are vermifuge.

Use. Treatment of impure blood, overheated blood, fevers, headache, anaemia, rickets. For high blood-pressure, diabetes.

Dose. One handful or more eaten as a salad, taken once or twice daily. For external use, pulp up the raw herb and apply where needed, binding into position with a damp cotton cloth. A teaspoonful of seeds every morning cures 'worms'.

QUEEN-OF-THE-MEADOW (*Eupatorium purpureum*. Corymbiferae). Found on low-lying land, likes damp soil. Leaves are medium, lance-shaped. Flowers are purple, tubular, growing in corymbs. The roots are the medicinal part used, and they are rather bitter, emitting when sliced an 'old-hay' smell.

This plant is the popular 'Joe-pie' of the American pioneer days, and a favourite of the American Indians. Its botanical name recalls a king of remote times, its common name, 'Joe-pie', is that of an Indian medicine-man. Formerly it was used in most American homes as a valued remedy against rheumatism and backache, ailments typical of those times of strenuous physical work and primitive housing conditions. Another common name of this plant is 'Gravel-root', on account of its healing effects on the kidneys and bladder and power in removing gravel and other deposits from the urinary system.

Use. Treatment of all rheumatic complaints, all ills of the joints including aching or sprained back. For all strains and sprains, and for treatment of pulled ligaments and tendons, disorders of the urinary system, and for removal of gravel and stones, treatment of inflamed bladder, scanty urine, burning urine, also dropsy. Soothing to the nerves, for neuralgia, headache, diabetes. An old remedy for gout.

132

Dose. Make a Standard brew of the finely sliced root. Take two tablespoons morning and night.

QUINCE (*Pyrus cydonia*. Rosaceae). I am considering this more as a shrub than a tree, as it is a shrub in its wild form. Quince happens to be a favourite of mine, owing to its valuable medicinal powers. The shrub is found in woodlands and cultivated in orchards and gardens. Leaves are the typical apple-tree form, of greyish green. Flowers are rose-form, large, very pink and sweetly scented. The fruits are large, pear-shaped, turning very hard, and yellow-brown when ripe. The fruit is the medicinal part; it is febrifuge, soothing, cooling. The seeds yield a valuable lotion when brewed. The inner side of the peel of the fruit has healing powers and is much used by Spanish gypsies and others for this purpose. The brewed peel is a hair tonic, and is used as a hair lotion in Arabian countries and is likewise valued as a hair grower for the manes and tails of the valued Arabian thoroughbred horses.

Use. The fruits as a raw pulp for treatment of diarrhoea, dysentery, haemorrhage of the bowels, and for venereal diseases (used internally and externally. Externally as a hair tonic — the brewed peel of the fruit). The brew also used to cleanse all discharging organs of the body. For all kinds of eye troubles, including general inflammation, ulcers, cysts and styes. The raw juice is also a hair tonic, and should be massaged into the scalp. Use the diluted juice, with a little lemon juice added, as a throat gargle; it is excellent for sore or relaxed throats; was once much used by singers to strengthen their voices.

Dose. One or two fruits, raw, grated, to be taken daily. Flavour with lemon juice and sweeten with honey. For those who cannot tolerate the rather coarse flesh of the quince, the fruit can be gently heated in sufficient water to cover, and cooked gently until soft, then sweetened with honey. Give a half cupful of the pulped fruit twice daily. A speedy remedy for griping stomach and intestinal pains is a teaspoon of quince juice with two powdered cloves, taken every few hours. The cooked, sieved fruit, reboiled with much sugar and half a lemon to every cupful of fruit, makes *Carne de membrillo*, the famous quince meat, a favourite of the Spanish people and of the Sephardic Jews, a tonic sweetmeat.

Dose. Make a Standard brew of the finely sliced fruit. Take two tablespoons morning and night.

RAGWORT (*Senecio Jacobaea*. Compositae). Found on waste land and in fields: loving the sun. The presence of ragwort is generally a sign of poor land. Leaves are finely cut, yellowish green. Flowers are starry, bright yellow, pungently aromatic. Very attractive to butterflies. The American Indian herbalists called this plant 'Squaw-weed', because of the use that Indian women made of it as a cure for all the ailments peculiar to their sex. However, since many herbalists have noted that ragwort can cause quite severe digestive upsets (I have observed this also in cattle when they have eaten too freely of ragwort) I advise its *external use only*. The flowers of ragwort have important forces which magnetize and remove deep-seated impurities, and which also dissolve swellings.

Use. Treatment of all skin ailments, gatherings, inflamed areas, tumours — soft and hard — and all types of swellings. Also boils, abscesses, whitlows.

Dose. External. Two handfuls of the flowers made into a Standard brew. Use hot and apply to the affected area, as fomentation or in massage.

RASPBERRY (*Rubus idaeus*. Rosaceae). Found in woodlands and in shady hedgerows. It likes water. Leaves are typical rose-form, thorny, with silver undersides. Flowers are also rose-form, pure white, with prominent stamens. Stems are bending and thorny. The fruits are a brilliant red, darkening when ripe, and very juicy. Raspberries are also widely cultivated in gardens, but the cultivated plant loses much of its medicinal powers, though still valuable. The wild raspberry is one of the most potent of all herbs and is not affected by mosaic disease which often attacks the cultivated species. Therefore when using cultivated plants, care must be taken to see that they are disease-free. The foliage of the raspberry plant possesses a very active principle, named *fragrine*. *Fragrine* has a special influence on the female organs of reproduction, especially on the muscles of the pelvic region and on the uterus. It is used as a female tonic throughout pregnancy and also during labour if any difficulty is encountered. It is also used to bring down retained afterbirth. It is an acclaimed remedy for sterility in male and female. It will relieve morning sickness. The whole plant also has other independent medicinal properties.

Use. The foliage and fruits as an aid to easy childbirth, for health of the mother and embryo. It would be rare for a gypsy woman to go through pregnancy without having taken raspberry leaf tea from the first weeks of knowledge of conception. And the true nomad gypsy gives birth to her children with the ease of the wild vixen.

In difficult labour, or afterwards to bring down retained afterbirth, strong drinks of raspberry-leaves tea, with a teaspoon of crushed ivy leaves to every two teaspoons of raspberry leaves, is given every two or three hours. This treatment has been successful when the more popular ergot (of rye) has failed. Add honey to give the patient extra strength. Is also helpful against frigidity and barrenness in men and women. Indeed, wild raspberry foliage and shoots are a well-known tonic for stallions and bulls.

The astringent properties of wild raspberry are employed to advantage in the treatment of dysentery and diarrhoea, especially the summer diarrhoea and fever of infants. Also used as a strengthening application (externally) for prolapsed uterus.

The ripe fruits are eaten as a general tonic, as a nervine, to supply readily assimilable iron, as a remedy for paleness, anaemia, fretfulness, general lack of energy.

Dose. Eat as many of the ripe fruits as desired, as often as possible.

Of the foliage, make a Standard brew and drink a large cupful on rising every morning during pregnancy. Drink a small cupful morning and night for other treatments. As a douche use the Standard brew cold. Also cold, a gargle for sore throats.

REED (the Great Reed) (*Arundo phragmites*, *Arundo donax*. Gramineae). Found by rivers and lakes and in ditches. The *culms*, blades, of this reed grow six feet high and even taller. Their inner white pith is medicinal, being a remedy for ailments of bladder and kidneys, and useful in treatment of dropsy.

Use. For all urinary ailments, lymphatic ailments, dropsy, goitre. Externally the pulped *culms* are applied to aching feet and joints and give much relief.

Dose. Extract the white inner pith by peeling the reeds, and eat a tablespoonful, raw, three times daily.

RHUBARB or WILD RHUBARB (*Rheum palmatum* or *Rheum rhaporticum*. Polygonaceae). Wild, it is found on waste land. Widely cultivated in gardens. Leaves are very large, umbrella-like, of rough texture, solitary and borne on very thick, fleshy, rose-hued stalks, which are edible, also medicinal. The leaves themselves are rank and not edible, as they possess some poisonous properties. The root is the most medicinal part and supplies one of the best aperients known to the herbalist. In small doses the root acts in a contrary way and will ease diarrhoea. The root has two unique substances, *binalate of potassium* and *rhubarbrin*, these are the secret of its medicinal virtues.

Use. Treatment of constipation in all forms including chronic, also diarrhoea, dysentery. An excellent laxative for infants on account of its smooth and mild action and because it is also tonic to the bowels. Treatment of headache, jaundice and all liver troubles. To reduce distended stomach in children, also for anaemia. For biliousness, lack of appetite, bad breath, colitis.

Dose. Eat a few of the raw young stems frequently as a bowel tonic and mild laxative. Take as much as desired of the lightly cooked stems and hearts, flavoured with lemon juice, sweetened with honey or sugar, for the purposes given above.

For a strong purge take the prepared rhubarb, obtainable from pharmacies, from ten to thirty grains of the prepared root, dose varying according to age and weight of person, but in any case over-dose is harmless. As a laxative from eight to twelve grains. As a tonic three to six grains. Of syrup of rhubarb take one teaspoon up to one dessertspoon. Take this prepared rhubarb in the early morning, on an empty stomach.

ROCK ROSE (*Cistus villosus*. Cistaceae). Found on dry, rocky, soil, on hillsides and banks. A sun-loving plant. Leaves are dark. Flowers like small single roses, frail, petals more square, prominent stamens: colour varied. This is an aromatic and astringent plant, yielding a valuable oil. It is one more of the short list of plants which herbalists consider beneficial in treatment of cancer. It has internal and external uses.

Use. As a gargle for sore and ulcerated throats. Treatment of venereal diseases. Considered good for infants, to cure their fears and give them courage. As a remedy for trembling. These last two uses are related to the rock rose's legendary reputation as a plant endowed with powers over the mind and spirit.

Dose. Of the oil two to three drops taken on a lump of sugar. Of the plant a Standard brew of leaves and/or flowers, used internally and externally. Internally a tablespoon three times daily.

For children (and for adults, if desired) an ancient remedy for timidity involves steeping flowers of rock-rose in sunlight and moonlight for two or three days, using preferably a shallow glass dish. At early morning and before bedtime, a tea-spoonful of the dish's contents is taken.

ROSE (BRIAR) (*Rose species*. Rosaceae). Found in hedge-rows and woodlands. Leaves are of rose form, with fine prickles. Flowers, large, pink or creamy, sweetly scented. Fruits are large, hard, red (hips). All species of rose, including the garden species, are a valuable tonic for the whole system and especially good for the heart.

They are a gentle astringent and slightly laxative. The fruits are also gently laxative. They are very vitamin-rich, especially in vitamin C, cooling to the blood, and of much benefit for cure of female ailments. The root was once advocated as a cure for rabies, and this is the possible reason for the name of one species of wild rose, *Rosa canina*, dog-rose. The ancient Celts used to employ this species of rose against infected wolf-bites, as treatment for themselves and for their domestic animals. The petals of the strongly scented species of garden rose, in particular the dark red roses, make a much valued sweetmeat in the Orient; it is also found in Provence. Also a syrup is made. The Turks prepare and sell a very valuable concentrated essence of roses, known as *attar* of roses.

Use. Treatment of catarrh, diarrhoea, haemorrhages. All female ailments, including leucorrhoea, metritis, threatened miscarriage. (The essential oil of roses is an active heart and brain tonic, and also a tonic for the ovaries and uterus.) Petals of the white rose make a soothing lotion, cooling and astringent, for sore or strained eyes.

Dose. Two dessertspoons of rose petals, pounded until softened and then taken in honey. Take in the early morning. Fruits: take six to eight fruits daily, either eaten raw or made into a tea and sweetened with honey. The fruits should be gently boiled until soft, when taken as a tea. Drink a small cupful morning and night. Oil: a few drops on a lump of sugar.

To make *confiture of red roses* (Turkish recipe): For every pound of freshly gathered red rose petals, take one pound of cane sugar, and three tablespoons of honey, the juice of one lemon. First add the lemon juice to the sugar, and gently heat until dissolved, then slowly add the honey, and heat further. Only when all the sugar is melted, slowly add the rose petals. Boil gently for an hour or so, stirring frequently, until the mixture begins to harden well against the sides of the pan. When almost ready to take from the fire add about three drops of almond oil to every pound weight of the mixture, and further heat for a few minutes. The oil makes the rose *confiture* shiny and also set better. But do not use too much almond oil or it will interfere with the natural delicious taste of the roses; add only a few drops. Spoon out into clean warm jars, and cover securely, when cold. Make this delicacy of roses preferably in an enamel or steel pan to prevent burning.

ROSEMARY (*Rosmarinus officinalis.* Labiatae). Found in sandy and rocky places, on slopes of mountains and on cliff-sides; can root where there is scanty soil. Loves the sun, loves the dew. Leaves are small, dark, shiny, hard and very aromatic. Flowers are small, lipped, varying from white-silver to dark blue. The sea has given rosemary its name — *Ros Marinus*, dew of the sea. (As a herbalist, if my name could be associated with any plant I would choose rosemary. I use it more than any other plant and I love it most of all. As Johnny Appleseed planted apples, so I plant rosemary wherever I travel. My present garden in Galilee is filled with rosemary grown from mere slips heeled into the earth.) Rosemary is widely cultivated in gardens where it is not only valued for its pleasant scent and its medicinal and culinary use, but also for the protection against insect pests that it gives to neighbouring plants and orchard trees. Rosemary is one of the most important of the aromatics. It yields a camphorated type of dark green oil which has many medicinal uses. It is also a proved supreme heart tonic, one of the few powerful heart tonics which is not a drastic drug. The gypsies especially love rosemary, and in former days they used to peddle the world-over a preparation of flowering rosemary sprigs, known as 'The Queen of Hungary's Water', much valued as a cure-all for the ills of mankind and as a general beautifier for women. The Arabs also greatly value rosemary; one use they make of it is to sprinkle the dried powdered herb on the umbilical cord of new-born infants as an astringent and antiseptic treatment. Spanish peasants pound rosemary into common salt and consider this remedy as the finest of all wound cures: the Arabs also extol this wound remedy. Herdsmen encourage their flocks to pasture on rosemary because of the pleasant taste this plant imparts to the milk; it is equally good for nursing mothers, carrying the values of this herb through the milk-flow to the feeding infant.

Rosemary is another of the few cure-all herbs of the herbalist. Externally it is valued for hair treatments and as an insecticide.

Use. Treatment of all ailments of the heart, also as a general heart tonic. Treatment of high blood-pressure, headaches, all nervous ailments. (The gypsies hang sprigs of rosemary in their vans as a protection against evil forces, and recommend placing sprigs under the pillow to protect sleepers — especially infants and children — and to prevent nightmares. I used it for my children.)

139

For all female ailments, including threatened miscarriage. For impure blood, gastritis, torpid liver, obesity. Externally for wounds of all kinds, for bites and stings, as a powerful insecticide, and as a wash to strengthen and brighten the hair and to check unnatural falling of hair. Also in cooking to flavour and garnish. In ancient times, rosemary was used in French churches and cathedrals for perfume, by crushing underfoot.

Dose. A sprig or so can be eaten raw daily in the salad, also a few leaves added chopped finely, to sandwiches, white cheese, soups, omelettes. Also make a Standard brew and drink as a warm tea, sweetened with honey, frequently during the day and as a night-cap.

Rosemary blends well with wormwood or vervain, sage and lavender, to make a most powerful antiseptic drink, invaluable in treatment of fevers and blood disorders.

Externally. The Standard brew as a hair-lotion, or a few drops of the infused oil, rubbed into the scalp. As an external treatment for wounds, use the lotion, or the fresh herbs pounded into salt and sprinkled on wounds and sores. Or the fresh or dried herb alone, pounded into a powder and applied. As an insecticide, a teaspoon of the oil to a half-pint of light beer. Or apply the dried herb in fine powder form mixed with wormwood in equal amounts.

RUE (*Ruta graveolens.* Rutaceae). Found in mountainous and barren places: a sun-loving plant. Widely cultivated in gardens, especially in Oriental countries where it is grown to protect the household against all evils. Rue decreases in value when dried.

Leaves are much divided, flat of greyish colour, very strongly aromatic and bitter tasting. Flowers are greenish-yellow, small, also flat, pungent of scent, bitter tasting. Rue contains a peculiar principle called *rutin*, which is highly medicinal. It has been proved effective as a strengthener of the blood-vessels, nerves and glands. *Rutin* also imparts hardness to the bones, teeth and nails. Doubtless the many legendary beliefs concerning rue come from the benefits that it imparts to

140

those who use it. It was always a favoured herb of the high priests in ancient times, and is to this present day also a cherished herb of the Arabs because this is the only one which Mahomet is known to have blessed. Arabic literature tells that Mahomet was cured of a fatal illness by the use of rue, which was brought to him by the gypsies when all the other remedies of his doctors had failed and he was dying. Rue is a remarkable expeller of poisons. This herb is reputed to resist all contagious poisions. In Iraq it is used to overcome fears and to make humans brave and is eaten, in sprigs, together with raisins. Leaves flavour wine and olives; flowers used for fertility.

Use. Treatment of all nervous ailments including hysteria, epilepsy, convulsions in children, and (like rosemary) had an ancient reputation for curing insanity. Treatment of all women's ailments, including faulty menstruation, congestion of the uterus, extreme pains in pregnancy. Good for all ailments of the arteries and veins and for weakness and palpitations of the heart. Good for fevers, colic, worms, also for treatment of rabies. Small sprigs are infused in hot water, sweetened with honey, and given to infants with upset stomachs. Sprigs are also oiled and inserted into the anus of infants to remove worms at night, or to relieve blocked anus. Externally in dried powder form or as a lotion, for treatment of all skin parasites, including head lice: also for ringworm. As a lotion, for treatment of eye ailments.

Dose. The herb is a potent one, therefore dosage should be small. A small teaspoonful of the herb to a tall glass of water, prepare as a Standard brew; take two tablespoons twice daily. For eye ailments, including treatment of cataract, dissolve the rue flowers by placing in a shallow vessel in the sunlight, adding a little white wine to the water — a teaspoon of wine to a cup of water. Infuse the flowers for three days. Measure of rue flowers is one tablespoonful to a cup. (When no sunlight is available, then slow heating in an oven with open door will do.) Bathe the eyes several times daily with the rue flowers water.

Rue has long been used as an antidote to the bites of snakes. Suck out the poison or cut out with the point of a sharp knife, in the usual way. Infuse two ounces of fresh rue in a pint of beer, drink this and apply some frequently to the bitten area. Also apply the infusion externally to the area of the bite.

RYE-GRASS (*Lolium* (species). Graminaceae). Found on pasture-land and in cultivation. Leaves of typical grass-form, the glumes on the flowering spikes turn very dark when ripened, and when rubbed emit a rather sour smell which is typical of rye.

In ancient times it was believed that rye, because of its potency, would destroy the wheat crop if it seeded amongst it. Its name is from the Celtic, 'to destroy'.

This is a powerful cereal, very rich in vitamins and minerals, especially rich in iron, and supplies valuable roughage. It is principally a muscle-builder. It is the basic cereal of the hardy Russians and Scandinavians.

Use. As a cereal, makes very healthful bread and flat biscuits. Is muscle-building and non-fattening. A good general digestive and nerve tonic. Rye bread soaked in hot water makes a good drawing poultice for all types of swellings and cysts. The typical rye bread has caraway seeds mixed in with the rye flour when making the dough. Rye-bread has excellent keeping qualities and will last for several weeks.

SAFFLOWER (*Carthamus tinctorius*. Compositae). SAFFRON (*Crocus sativus*. Iridaceae). The safflower is the herb now under discussion. It is found mostly in Mediterranean countries, in its wild form, frequenting dry plains and hill slopes. Also widely cultivated in other lands, including England and America on account of the rich yellow dye that it yields. (*Tinctoris* of course, meaning dye — or woad.) Leaves are alternate, smooth and shining. Flowers are numerous, long, slender, of orange hue and with a pungent scent. Known also as Dyer's Saffron, the flowers yield two dyes, a bright yellow which can be extracted in water, and a vivid red extracted only by alcohol. This plant, considered an 'old-fashioned' remedy has many valuable medicinal powers, especially effective in treatment of fevers, and is considered a specific for scarlet fever, chicken-pox, measles and other eruptive diseases: it will

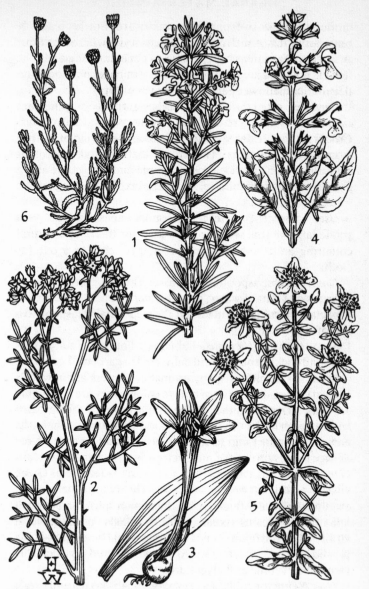

Plate 12. 1. Rosemary 2. Rue 3. Safflower (Saffron)
4. Sage 5. St. John's Wort 6. Santolina

produce profuse sweating when taken as a hot beverage. A generous pinch of saffron from crocus styles will colour flour and rice, saffron buns being once very popular in England. The flowers and seed are the parts used. It was once common practice to mix safflower petals with crocus saffron.

Carthamus tinctorius or 'Dyer's Saffron', is sometimes called False Saffron, to distinguish it from the saffron crocus, *Crocus sativus*, Iridaceae, which yields another kind of saffron from its dried stigmas. This crocus saffron is also used for colouring flour and rice, and is a tonic and a digestive aid, a proved remedy for jaundice. A pinch is taken in a glass of white wine.

Use. Treatment of fevers, irregular menstruation. As a gentle laxative (the seeds are also used for this). As a natural colouring and flavouring for cakes, rice, etc. As a dye for cloth.

Dose. A dessertspoon of the flowers heated gently in three-quarters of a pint of water, or half water and half milk. Take a wineglass morning and night. Of the seeds a half-teaspoon to a cup of hot water.

SAGE (*Salvia officinalis*. Labiatae). Found on sunny hillsides and rocky grounds, and cultivated in gardens. Leaves are oval, rather woolly, strongly aromatic. Flowers are in whorls and vary from silver to deep blue in colour, they are also highly aromatic. This is another of the major herbs of the herbalist and has been in the service of mankind since ancient times. Its name is from the Latin *salvere*, 'to be well' and 'to save'. A tea of sage tops is one of the most refreshing and beneficial available to mankind. The scent from sage tea is a feature of Greek villages as it is brewed in the cafés. This plant is believed to exert a beneficial influence over the human spirit, and to quell unnatural or vicious sexual desires. It will also restore normal virility when the failure is not due to venereal disease. Sage is a proved help in fevers, and is also a vermifuge and insecticide. A valued heart tonic and fever cure.

Use. A cure for colds, sore throats, coughs (as tea and gargle for such), sore and ulcerated mouths. All fevers, digestive ailments — especially flatulence and lack of appetite, constipation, obesity. To increase the milk yield and to give tonic properties to the milk. For all nervous ailments, including paralysis and mild mental derangement; to improve the memory. Externally the pulped herb, for all forms of wounds, sores, ulcers, to allay excessive bleeding. An effective hair-tonic, to stimulate growth, tone up the colour and act as a setting lotion, to remove dandruff. To deter moths, cockroaches and rodents from clothes closets. Also as an inhalation and in sweat baths. A teeth cleanser. And as a cheese flavour.

Dose. Make a Standard brew and take a cupful morning and night, sweetened with honey. As sage is a potent herb, a teaspoon of the herb to a half-pint of water is sufficient. Sage can also be infused in the sunlight without requiring fire-heat, to yield pleasantly flavoured and tonic water. Externally, use the Standard brew as a lotion. For clothes closets, tie the sage in bunches and place within. Sage is excellent as an inhalation for congestion of the nose and head, and placed in the water for steam baths, having been much used in this way by the ancient Mexicans.

The wild sage of Mexico and neighbour regions, *Salvia azurea grandiflora*, with its blue highly scented blossoms, is powerfully medicinal, so also is Red Sage, *Salvia colorata*, red sage being considered a 'cure-all', and especially good for ailments of the throat and lungs, including tuberculosis.

SAINT JOHN'S WORT (*Hypericum perforatum*. Hyperidaceae). Found along waysides and in woodlands. Prefers shady places. Leaves are multiform, frail, and peculiar for the bright specks covering them, which are oil glands. The flowers are terminal and held in leafy panicles. They are bright yellow, of poppy form, and have a crowd of silky prominent stamens. The plant possesses medicinal resins, also acids and a gum. The herb is astringent and soothing. The fresh flowers steeped in sun- or fire-warmed olive oil yield the famed Oil of Saint John's Wort, much used by the Crusader knights. The flowers combined with chamomile, and mixed into melted fat with some bees-wax added, give an ointment which is renowned for its pain quelling and healing properties. Saint John's Wort is said to protect the home against harm and loss; in former times much used in magic charms.

Use. Treatment of wounds and ulcers, internal and external. Also for haemorrhages, dysentery, diarrhoea, jaundice, earache, toothache, hysteria, and general nervousness, fainting fits, rheumatism, arthritis, worms, especially thread-worms. Externally for all wounds, eruptions, abrasions, blisters of all kinds, inflammations, rashes — including those from infectious ailments, such as scarlet fever and typhus. Also for burns and scalds.

Dose. Make a Standard brew and take two tablespoons three times daily. Externally use the Standard brew as a lotion. For the Oil of Saint John's Wort, steep one handful of the finely cut flowers in a half-pint of olive oil and heat gently (*see* Herbal oils). Apply the oil as a soothing rub. It will also deter insects.

SANICLE (*Sanicula mariandica*. Umbelliferae). Found in woods and thickets. Leaves are finely serrate and dark. Flowers are in umbels and are greenish white. The many barren flowerlets are stalkless. The plant derives its name from a word meaning 'to heal', because this is another intensely curative herb. A favourite of the Crusaders; they often painted pictures of sanicle on their shields. The promise concerning this plant is written as: 'to make whole and sound alle inwarde hurts and outwards woundes of man'. Not to be compared with 'American' and 'Yorkshire' sanicles.

Use. Treatment of all internal wounds, ulcers, haemorrhages.

As a remedy for stomach-ache and aches in the bowels. Treatment of inflamed lungs and tuberculosis. Externally, for all wounds and sores, sore throat, inflamed gums, treatment of rashes, erysipelas.

Dose. A weak tea, to be taken in doses of tablespoons before meals.

SANTOLINA (*Diotis maritima*. Compositae). Found on sea-cliffs. Also on wasteland and cultivated in gardens, being a common border herb. Leaves are grey, ferny in form, rather

146

woolly and highly aromatic. Flowers are small, yellow, button-form and also very aromatic. A very tonic, tangy tea herb.

Use. Finely minced, mixed into a pill with thick honey and used as a fever and worm remedy. Externally a strong brew as a wound herb. Infused in vinegar as a rheumatism rub. The flowers sun-infused in oil and vinegar yield a deep yellow oil which is a remedial rub for aches and pains and is also mildly insecticide. This herb, in muslin bags, is placed in linen and clothes closets against moths.

Dose. One teaspoon daily.

SCABIOUS (Field) (*Scabiosa arvensis*. Dipsacaceae). Found in fields and on banks. Also cultivated in gardens. Leaves are wavy and rather poppy-form. Flowers are solitary, rather daisy type, borne on round stems, usually purple colour, very honey-scented. A favourite of the gypsies, one of its names being 'Gypsy Rose'.

The whole herb is very blood-cleansing and antiseptic.

Use. Treatment of all skin ailments, all female ailments. Heart weakness and disease, in old times against venereal disease. (Internal dosing and external application.) Externally a brew of the roots will cure old sores and gatherings. A brew of the whole herb, including the root, thickened with borax, will remove dandruff from the head.

Dose. Infuse a handful of the flowers in a pint of wine. Take two tablespoons morning and night. External: Make a Standard brew of the roots and use cold.

SEA-HOLLY (*Eryngium maritimum*. Umbelliferae). Found along sea-coasts. Leaves are spiked, stiff, silver-grey with delicate blue-veins and tints. Flowers are terminal, dense, and of an intense blue, honey-scented. Rich in minerals and nerve-tonic properties. It is especially rich in silica. The Arabs eat the young shoots, lightly boiled. The roots are also edible and the Arabs candy them as a delicacy. The cut herb can be piled around trees to protect them against vermin.

Use. Treatment of liver ailments, chest ailments, glandular deficiencies and disorders, constipation. As a nerve tonic and general tonic.

147

Dose. One root lightly boiled or baked, finely sliced and eaten in the daily salad.

SEA-LAVENDER (*Statice limonium*. Plumbaginaceae). Found along muddy shores and on marshes. Leaves are finely pleated and broken edged, dry and membraneous. Flowers are also dry, in corymbose panicles, of a pale lavender colour and faintly honey-scented. They are sometimes flecked with white.

Its name is derived from the word 'to stop', and alludes to its strong astringent powers, used in treatment of wounds and to check dysentery. Statice was much used on the battle-fields of Britain in ancient days, and the gypsies use it still to stem bleeding.

Use. As an astringent wound herb, and to treat all forms of haemorrhage, treatment of dysentery, diarrhoea, bed-wetting.

Dose. Steep a handful of the flowers in a quart of cider, and take two tablespoons night and morning. (Cider is also an astringent in dysentery.) External use: merely crush the flowers and apply direct to wounds.

SENNA (*Cassis acutifolia*. Leguminosae). Found on open plains. Leaves are bean-like. Flowers pea-form of various colours, producing flat pods. Senna contains special acids, gums and sugars. It is one of the most powerful laxatives in the herbal kingdom and the one that I advise most often in my herbal treatments.

As a laxative it tones and restores the digestive system as well as very thoroughly cleansing it. The griping pains which are typical of treatment with senna are caused by the laxative breaking down hard adhesions in the bowels. These pains are only brief whilst the laxative is working, and can be much reduced by the addition of a pinch of powdered ginger to every cupful of the laxative infusion.

Use. Treatment of constipation, including chronic form. To cleanse the system during fasting and in all fevers. For catarrhal ailments, jaundice, obesity, faulty menstruation, worms.

Dose. For an adult person an average of eight to ten large senna pods (the kind sold in pharmacies under the name of

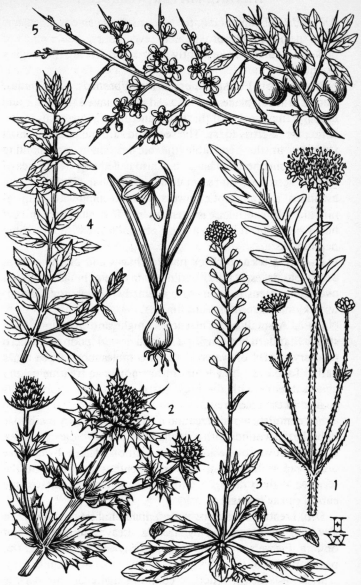

Plate 13. 1. Scabious 2. Sea Holly 3. Shepherd's Purse
4. Skullcap 5. Sloe 6. Snowdrop

Alexandrian Senna pods), to three-quarters cup of cold water. Soak the pods for approximately seven hours. Add a pinch of powdered ginger. Take nightly until the bowels are thoroughly clean.

SHEPHERD'S PURSE (*Capsella bursa-pastoris*. Cruciferae). Found in waste places and as weed in cultivated fields. Leaves are tiny, like the rest of this herb, and dark. Flowers also tiny, white, set in cross form. The seed pods are the distinguishing features, as they resemble the old-fashioned leather sling purses of shepherds. The herb is also called shepherd's heart, and the seed pods do resemble a heart in shape. It has strong astringent and antiseptic powers out of keeping with its insignificance. Its special use is as emergency first-aid where there is heavy bleeding. It is also a good general tonic with a pleasing peppery taste.

Use. Was used to check haemorrhages and bleeding from deep wounds, especially bleeding from nose or lungs. To lessen over-heavy menstruation. Also a remedy for diarrhoea, dysentery, kidney disorders, ear ailments.

Dose. A small handful chewed night and morning. Or a strong Standard brew, using a heaped dessertspoon of the herb to every cupful of water. Take two tablespoons three times daily. Take every few hours in haemorrhage treatment, and give a douche with the brew, used cold. Also apply cloths soaked in the cold brew.

For complete wound treatment, the French gypsy method is to bathe the wounds with a strong brew of the whole herb, then plug with clean cobwebs. I cannot define a 'clean cobweb', but I can report successes. Ear treatment: a teaspoon of the warmed brew is dropped into both ears, and the base of the ears is gently massaged.

SKULL-CAP (*Scutellaria galericulata*. Labiatae). Found in low-lying meadows and by streams. Leaves are crenate and oblong. Flowers are rather large, downy and bright blue. The peculiar form of the calyx gives the plant its Latin name (from *scutella* — shield). Another common name of this herb is 'Mad-dog weed', giving indication of the herb's powerful

150

sedative powers and its use in former days in rabies. The herb is indeed a supreme nerve remedy and has cured cases of insanity which no other medicine had improved. Also used to give natural sleep to morphine addicts, especially when combined with lime-blossom, catnip and hops.

Use. Treatment of all nervous disorders, including fits, epilepsy, convulsions, chorea, delirium tremens. Also for general excitability, wakefulness, headache. Treatment of bites of poisonous insects. Also a cure for sterility, used internally and externally (as a lotion or douche).

Dose. A Standard brew of the whole herb. Take a wineglass morning and night, sweetened with honey. Externally, use the Standard brew.

SLOE (*Prunus spinosa*. Rosaceae). Found in hedgerows and copses. Leaves are small, plum-like and dark. Flowers are white, rose-form, fragrant, and give small, dark, plum-like fruits which are very sharp and strongly astringent. The flowers are amongst the first to appear in the early spring; 'blackthorn' blossom whitens the hedges sometimes before the last snows have gone. The flowers, fruits and bark are all used. The flowers are gently laxative and vermifuge. The fruits are a tonic astringent and the bark is antispasmodic and sedative. Gypsies ripen the fruits, and render them sweeter, by burying them in straw-lined pits deep in the ground, for several months.

Use. The flowers: treatment of all fevers, blood disorders, constipation, lack of appetite, worms. The fruits: all fevers, skin ailments, dropsy. The bark: Nervous disorders, twitchings, whooping-cough.

Dose. Of the flowers: eat a handful every morning. Of the fruits: eat three or four, grated into honey to lessen their bitterness and the unpleasant tartness in the mouth. Take in the early morning. Of the bark: shave finely and make a brew of one tablespoon to a half-pint of cold water. Bring to the boil, simmer for several minutes, allow to steep for four hours, sweeten with honey and take a tablespoon of the brew three times daily before meals.

SNOWDROP (*Galanthus nivalis*. Amaryllidaceae). Found in shady and damp places, especially woodlands. Leaves are slender, narrow, stalkless. Flowers are drooping, white, frail, lily-like, marked with green honey guides, fragrant. Flowers and bulbs used, externally only. A lotion from crushed flowers whitens the skin.

Use. Treatment of frost-bite, chilblains.

Dose. Slice up three or four bulbs, steep them in half a pint of light beer, apply as a lotion. For frost-bite add a heaped teaspoon of powdered cayenne pepper to every half-pint of snowdrop beer. A friction also for circulatory ailments.

SOAPWORT (*Saponaria officinalis*. Caryophyllaceae). Found along roadsides, also likes to grow close to cottages, where it is welcomed on account of its pleasant and fragrant flowers and also for its usefulness. Leaves are oval, shiny, fragile. Flowers are pale pink, crinkled, usually double, and sweetly scented. Common name, especially in America, is 'Bouncing Bet'.

This plant yields a peculiar mucilaginous juice, which in water or alcohol resembles soap in solution, and can be used instead of soap. It is the element *saponin* that imparts the foaming and cleansing properties.

Even in modern times, this plant is much used in expensive toilet articles, such as hair shampoos and hand lotions. And when the way of life of the American Indians is discussed it is commonly mentioned that the Indians used for their washing a lathery substance produced from the leaves of a plant: it is 'Bouncing Bet'. The roots are also used to remove stains and for washing woollens.

Herbalists employ this herb internally in treatment of liver ailments and asthma. Personally I would advise external use only.

Use. Treatment of inflamed and discharging areas of the body, including leucorrhoea, gonorrhoea, erysipelas. Also as a rub for stiff joints, rheumatism, arthritis and cramps.

Dose. A decoction of the finely shaved root, either in water as a Standard brew, or a tablespoonful steeped in light beer overnight. Employ cold as a lotion, douche or rub.

152

SORREL (*Rumex acetosa*. Polygonaceae). Found on waste land and in fields. Leaves are arrow-shaped and very acid-tasting, flowers are reddish and grow in tall spikes: sometimes the flower spikes are of green or brown colour. The whole plant is very cooling, its acid quality being beneficial to the human body. The leaves are used to curdle milk and for junket-making, the leaves and stems being well crushed to express their juice, or a strong decoction is made from the leaves, using some heat, and that can also be used in junket-making, etc.

Also called sour-grass it is an old-fashioned salad herb; a few leaves are added to the salad for their blood-cooling effect; also they may be cooked in the same way as spinach and served with a pinch of salt and a little butter.

The oxalic acid, formerly known as 'salts of Sorrel' was once used as a stain-remover, especially for difficult stains such as iron-mould. This acid is in all parts of the plant.

Sorrel is also highly medicinal and is used with benefit for blood, kidney and liver disorders, and for all fevers.

Use. Treatment of impure blood, boils, eczema, and all fevers. Also inflammation of the kidneys, gravel in kidneys, jaundice and all liver complaints, for internal ulcers of the digestive tract or elsewhere. Externally: to cleanse sweaty skin, and to cure all types of skin eruptions and festering sores. A cold poultice is good for tumours, abscesses and boils.

Dose. Eat four or five leaves once or twice daily. Eat further as a boiled vegetable. Or make a Standard brew and drink several tablespoons three times daily, sweetened with honey. Externally, apply the fresh leaves pounded into a pulp and macerated in milk or water. Make also a poultice of the fresh leaves, use cold.

SOUTHERNWOOD (*Artemisia abrotanum*. Compositae). Found on sunny hillsides. Leaves are conspicuous, hoary, feathery, grey-green and of sweet and pungent scent. Flowers are in slender racemes and of green-yellow colour. Also much cultivated in herb gardens. The whole plant contains a bitter principle in the form of an oil called *absinthol*, which possesses highly antiseptic properties, is also vermifuge and insecticide

153

like other herbs of the *Artemisia* group. Artemis, or Diana the huntress, was the Greek goddess who watched over women and children and guarded them at the time of birth.

Use. Treatment of all female ailments and ailments of newborn infants, complaints of bladder and kidneys, as a vermifuge. Externally as a hair-wash and lotion, especially good against diseases of the scalp and parasites. Also to cleanse the skin of lice and their eggs. To keep moths and other harmful insects from clothing and linen.

Dose. A Standard brew of the leaves. Take a small wineglass morning and night: sweeten with honey. Externally: use a stronger brew, or use a powder from the dried herb. To repel moths, lay sprigs of the plant amongst clothing.

SOW-THISTLE (*Sonchus arvensis*. Compositae). Found on waste land, in gardens and in cultivated fields. Leaves have triangular lobes and prickly edges. Flowers are small, yellow, and of thistle-form. The whole plant is very refrigerant and is therefore used in ailments of the blood and in fevers. Legend says that hunted hares when hard-pressed by hounds, will stay to snatch a few mouthfuls of this herb to cool their blood and succour their bursting hearts. A common name for this plant is 'Hare's-Lettuce'. Incidentally this plant is also a remedy for palpitations of the heart. The whole plant is very rich in minerals. The young hearts are eaten as a salad herb by gypsies everywhere and by peasants of the Swiss and French Alps, also by the Arabs.

Use. Treatment of all fevers, skin disorders, acid stomach, disorders of the intestinal tract. To allay heart palpitations, heart tonic, and for anaemia. The white milk expressed from the leaves and stems makes a good application for sunburn.

Dose. A handful of the young leaves to be eaten daily. Give more often for treatment of heart disorders. If the leaves have coarsened, trim off the prickly edges.

SPEEDWELL (*Veronica officinalis*. Scrophulariaceae). Found in pastures and copses. Leaves are tiny, rough, serrated. Flowers are small, delicate, pale blue and marked with a white eye. This is one more minute herb which has remarkable medicinal powers out of proportion with its size. Speedwell removes excess mucus from the body, soothes all internal tissues, and provides a tonic tea much used by the gypsies everywhere.

Use. Treatment of cough, bronchial asthma, pulmonary catarrh, pleurisy, tuberculosis, ulcerated lungs. Also dysentery, jaundice.

As a tea the herb is highly tonic and blood-cleansing and a stimulant of the gastric juices. Externally, for all skin inflammations, eruptions, ulcers, rashes. For all eye ailments, to improve the sight.

Dose. A handful of the herb eaten raw once daily. Or make a Standard brew and drink as a tea, a wineglass morning and night, at least three times daily in serious lung troubles. Externally: the brew is used as a gargle for relieving catarrh, and as a cold lotion for application to the skin and for bathing the eyes.

SPHAGNUM MOSS (*Sphagnum cymbifolium*. Musci). Found in damp places, especially peaty moors. In form this handsome moss is rather like edelweiss. Leaves are soft, ferny, and peculiar for their water-storing properties. Their colour is greenish yellow, sometimes orange-stained through the high iodine content. It is a plant of the *Bryophyta* group, which is between the ferns and the seaweeds. Its chief use is as a surgical dressing, as it is able to absorb many times its own weight of whatever moisture it is in contact with, when itself rendered into a dry state — which is easily done by gathering and exposing it to sunlight and wind. (When drying sphagnum, care must be taken that it is not carried away by the wind, for it dries to a feathery lightness.) It is very antiseptic, cooling and soothing, and makes excellent bandage material. Sphagnum moss, partly dried and then soaked in a brew of a strongly antiseptic herb such as garlic, elder blossom, wormwood, rue, etc., is much used by gypsies and American Indians for skin and wound treatments. Soaked in beer for burns and scalds. The American Indian women also used this moss as sanitary pads and as lining for the portable cradles of their infants, who need not

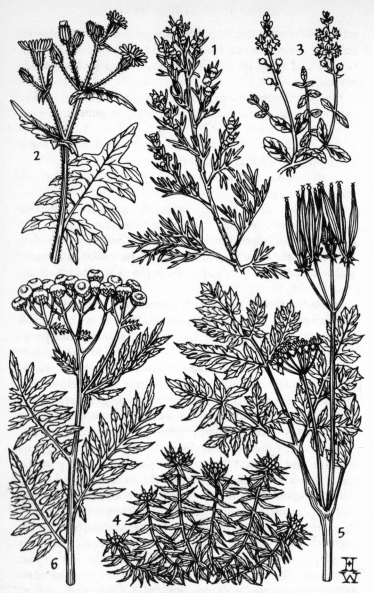

Plate 14. 1. Southernwood 2. Sow-Thistle 3. Speedwell
4. Sphagnum Moss 5. Sweet Cecily 6. Tansy

therefore wear uncomfortable napkins. Sphagnum moss is a base of that important fuel, peat.

STONECROP or BITING STONECROP (*Sedum acre*. Crassulaceae). Found on rocky and sandy soil, especially in coastal areas. Also grows on old walls. Leaves are in rosettes and are succulent and upstanding. Flowers are also somewhat succulent, starry, yellow in colour. It is employed in nervous ailments and externally for obstinate gatherings in the skin tissues including those of a malignant nature.

Use. Treatment of epilepsy, chorea, convulsions, hysteria. Externally as a lotion or salve (the herb pounded into melted cold cream or vegetable fat) for old swellings, abscesses, boils, cysts, tumours.

STRAWBERRY or WILD STRAWBERRY (*Fragaria vesca*. Rosaceae). Found on shady banks and in woodlands, likes a rich soil. Also widely cultivated in gardens — private and market. Leaves are dark green, glossy, fan shaped. Flowers, white, rose-form, with prominent yellow centre; fruits are small, round, red, very juicy berries. The whole plant is very refrigerant, and also highly minerals-rich and antiseptic. The fruits are prized above all others by the American Indians, and are cooling, strengthening, healing, also mildly vermifuge. The leaves and root also are medicinal, very cooling and mildly laxative. The leaves are a proved aid in preventing abortion, they also regulate faulty menstruation. They make an excellent tea for the feverish.

Use. Fruits and leaves (similar). Treatment of impure blood, thin blood, anaemia, lowered vitality, feeble nerves, lack of appetite. For all bowel disorders, stomach disorders, liver diseases. Treatment of fevers, undue sweating, abortion, menstrual irregularities. The fruit alone is a powerful nerve tonic. The fruit may be used externally for cleansing the teeth and for removing discoloration and other blemishes from the skin.

Dose. Of the leaves, make a tea, Standard method. Take a small wineglass morning and night. Use the brew externally as a soothing lotion for eczema, sore eyes, styes on the eyelids. The fruit: eat as much as desired as often as desired. The season of cultivated garden strawberries is a short one; wild woodland strawberries enjoy a longer season and are richer in iron. Eat as many as possible and preserve some in melted honey with a little lemon juice added. There are some people who after eating strawberries, develop 'Strawberry Rash'; this is only evidence of the cleansing action of the strawberries, driving excess acid from the system more speedily than the body can expel it by other channels.

SUMMER SAVORY (*Satureja hortensis*. Labiatae). Found on banks in sunny places, likes a sandy soil. Leaves are small, narrow, fan shaped, very numerous; flower heads are thick clusters, calyx grey, petals dark purple, hooded. The whole plant is highly aromatic and has a scent rather like a mingling of lavender and apples: indeed a summer savory! In use, is similar to most of the aromatics, especially of the Labiatae family, as an antiseptic and general tonic. Much used also as a tonic for those who are frigid or lacking in virility.

Used as a pot herb, to flavour salads, vinegar, soups. Can also be placed among clothing to deter destructive insects.

Use. Treatment of all fevers, especially those of an infectious kind. To sweeten the breath, stomach and intestines. As a nervine, also as a tonic for the reproductive system; to regulate irregular menstruation. Treatment of wind in infants, diarrhoea, colds.

As a flavouring and pot herb.

Dose. A few sprigs eaten in salad or soups. Or make a Standard brew and take a small cupful morning and night. Flowering sprigs are placed in clothes cupboards and linen closets to repel moths.

SWEET CECILY (*Myrrhis odorata*. Umbelliferae). Found in hedges, on edges of woods, also on mountain-sides, cultivated in gardens. The leaves are pale green, feathery and with a most sweet scent. Flowers are white and in large umbels. The whole plant is useful to the herbalist, from the roots to the seeds. The American Indians eat the pungent seeds and roots, and use the roots as a bait to catch wild horses. The plant is a general tonic and appetizer and is mildly laxative, especially the seeds. The foliage is put into linen closets to impart a pleasant scent to the contents. In France the dried plant is used for stuffing pillows.

Use. As a tonic cordial, to restore appetite, strengthen the nerves. The roots, steamed and mashed, as a poultice for boils.

Dose. Make a Standard brew of the foliage. Take a wine-glass morning and night. One or two roots, or some seeds (salted) can be roasted and eaten.

SWEET FLAG (CALAMUS) (*Acorus calamus.* Araceae). Found in marshy places and alongside streams and rivers; it will also grow in quite deep water. Its leaves are distinctive, being reed-like but having wavy edges. The flowers are rush-like, in blunt spikes, yellow, sometimes tending to rusty brown. A common name is Sweet Sedge, for it is a scented plant, especially the root. This rhizome has inner tissues of a pinky white shade, and is of spongy texture and very aromatic. It is rich in food values and is highly medicinal. The chief value of the root of sweet flag is its influence over the whole digestive system, sweetening, purifying and strengthening, improving the digestive juices and quelling fermentation. Will correct over-acid condition of the whole body.

Use. As a nutritive tonic, for invalids, tubercular cases, and in the weaning of infants.

Treatment of gastritis, dysentery, mild and chronic constipation, lack of appetite and general debility. Externally for sores, wounds, inflammations, burns and scalds.

Dose. A small teaspoon of the powdered root mixed with two tablespoons of lightly roasted wheaten flour, and mixed into a gruel with milk, sweetened with honey. Take a spoonful or more at midday and evening, after meals. More can be taken if liked. For weaning infants give twice daily.

SWEET GALE (*Myrica gale.* Myricaceae). Found on moorlands and on boggy wastes. Leaves are greyish, pointed, sweetly scented. Flowers are pinkish, and the fruits are waxy berries of a bright orange colour. The New Forest gypsies taught me the use of this charming plant. They gather the leaves for the making of home-brewed beer. In remote times leaves of sweet gale (or bog-myrtle as the Forest gypsies call it) were often used along with hops in the brewing of beer.

The plant is a general tonic and a wound herb. Wild deer and ponies seek it out for its tonic properties.

Use. Treatment of general debility, weak nerves, lack of appetite, poor sleep. To remedy mental depression, lassitude, poor memory. Externally the leaves are applied as a hot poultice to cauterize wounds.

Dose. A Standard brew of the leaves. Take a wineglass in the early morning, sweeten with honey to counteract bitterness. Externally: pulp up several handfuls of leaves, heat slowly in a little hot water or beer until softened, apply hot to the wound.

TANSY (*Tanacetum vulgare.* Compositae). Found along roadsides and on waste lands. Leaves are dark, ferny and of pungent scent. Flowers are small, of brilliant yellow, in peculiar flat discs, borne in clusters, of pungent scent. The whole plant has a camphor-type odour and is hot and peppery to taste. A highly medicinal plant, and a favourite of the English gypsies who frequently name their children Tansy. It is one of the most mineral-rich of all herbs and contains many remarkable substances, including stearin, gallic acid, gum, precipitate of lime, bitter resin. It yields a bright yellow colouring matter which in former days was used in confectionery, for tansy buns and tansy sugar rock. It is almost a cure-all herb having so many medicinal values. It is tonic, soothing, nervine, vermifuge, and good for external treatments of swellings, tumours, etc.

Use. An excellent general tonic, used in convalescence from enervating diseases; against failing appetite, nausea, morning sickness, threatened abortion. Also all fevers, most digestive complaints, kidney ailments, jaundice, dropsy. To cure menstrual disorders, arteries and strengthen the veins, a remedy for varicose veins, also for high blood-pressure, heart weaknesses. Externally also for application to enlarged, knotted or varicose veins. Treatment of all swellings, bruises, earache, toothache, styes and eye inflammation.

Dose. This is a strong herb and can only be taken in small doses. Make a Standard brew using only one small teaspoon of the finely cut herb to every cup of water. Take a tablespoon of this brew three times daily before meals. Externally: use the lotion hot, wringing out a cotton cloth in the brew and applying where needed, renewing the hot cloths as they cool. The dried powdered flower heads can be added to flour for colouring and giving a tangy flavour. Use one dessertspoon of the flowers to every pound of flour.

TEASEL (*Dipsacus fullorum*. Dipsacaceae). Found in waste places and on hedge-banks. Not a common plant. Leaves are large and serrated, stems of the plant are very prickly (to prevent theft, by undesirable insects, of the precious water held in the hollows of the upper conate leaves). Flowers somewhat resemble the thistle heads of the Compositae order, and are in long, oval, tightly-packed heads of pale purple shading to white. The flower heads are held in a thorny receptacle once much used in dressing cloth, the hooked scales being admirably placed by nature for that very purpose. The plant derives its name from a word meaning 'to be thirsty', alluding to the water stored in the leaves which is used to trap winged insects, which the plant absorbs.

Use. This teasel herb provides a wonderful remedy for eye ailments and for applying to styes, whitlows on fingers, and for erasing wrinkles from the face. I learnt the use of teasel water from Somerset gypsies.

Dose. Not specific. Use as much teasel water as one is fortunate enough to find and collect!

THRIFT (*Armeria vulgaris*. Plumbaginaceae). Found along seashores and on mountain-sides. Leaves are short, reedy, grooved. Flowers are in round heads of pale pink, honey-scented flowerets set amongst brown scales. Flowers are sometimes almost white. The flowers are a fine bee-food, they are tonic and restoring to man.

Use. Nervine, tonic, as a tea to alleviate mental depression.

Dose. Standard brew of the flowers. Take a wineglass once daily.

THYME (*Thymus serpyllum* and *Thymus vulgaris*. Labiatae). Found on heaths and on sunny banks. Leaves are small, flat, dark green and very sweetly aromatic. Flowers are in whorls, and are tiny, lilac in colour, and also very aromatic. This is a most valuable plant and has been used in medicine since the very earliest days of herbal treatment. The plant is a powerful antiseptic and general tonic. It yields an essential oil which accounts for its antiseptic virtues and which is also a good vermifuge. This oil is called thymol and is found in many orthodox preparations such as disinfectants, dentifrices, hair lotions. The dried and powdered herb provided the well-known condiment of the Arabs, called Za'atar. The powdered thyme is mixed with roasted sesame and coriander seeds and salt, and that is Za'atar, eaten with bread. In the Balearic isles is used to preserve dried fruits.

Use. Treatment of all digestive complaints, including inflammation of the liver, bad breath, flatulence. Treatment of whooping-cough, sore throat, asthma, sinus ailments, rickets. Treatment of all nervous derangements, including hysteria, nervous indigestion, nightmares, headaches. To control excessive menstrual flow, expel retained afterbirth, treatment of inflamed or diseased uterus, mastitis and all swellings of the breasts. A safe remedy for worms, even in infants. Used to promote perspiration in fevers.

Externally: as a hot fomentation for abscesses, boils, and all kinds of swellings and gatherings.

Dose. Eat some sprigs of thyme raw, fresh, in the daily salad, rubbing the leaves off the stems. Prepare the dried powdered herb, the Za'atar, and eat this with olive oil on slices of bread. Make a Standard brew and take a wineglass morning and night.

TOAD-FLAX (*Linaria vulgaris*. Scrophulariaceae). Found in waste places, fields and amongst growing corn. Leaves are small and flat, flowers are in racemes of yellow and orange marked white and are of familiar snapdragon form. This herb has powerful dissolvent properties, and is therefore used to treat obstructions in all parts of the body. It also provides one of the best jaundice remedies known to the herbalist.

Use. Treatment of jaundice. Obstructions in the intestines, kidneys, bladder. Lymphatic disorders, dropsy.

Dose. A Standard brew of the whole herb. Take two tablespoons three times daily.

TRAVELLER'S JOY. *See* VIRGIN'S BOWER.

VALERIAN (*Valeriana officinalis.* Verbenaceae). Found on sunny banksides and on old walls. Its leaves are bright green, opposite, compound, shiny. Flowers are in corymbs of rose or white. The root is the medicinal part of this important herb and its healing virtues have given Valerian the common name of 'All-heal'.

The roots are perennial and should be allowed to be at least two years of age before being lifted. The taste of the root is rather nauseous and its odour unpleasant. This scent makes the valerian useful as a rat bait, as they come to it eagerly.

There is *valerianic* acid in the roots. Also starch, balsamic resin, mucilage, albumen, a substance *valerianin*, and many minerals; particularly there is a rich silica content. All these ingredients of the root make it a most important nerve remedy. Of valerian, the American Indian herbalists believe that if epileptic fits will not yield to this herb they are incurable.

In over-large doses, valerian causes headache, mental agitation including delusions and much restlessness. It is said that Hitler was a valerian addict. Properly used, valerian is a supreme remedy for all types of nerve trouble, is good for the heart, useful in fevers. Externally is a soothing and strengthening agent.

Use. Treatment of epilepsy, hysteria, chorea, convulsions in children, paralysis. Also for chronic constipation, worms, malaria and other recurrent fevers. Externally valerian (especially the expressed oil in solution in alcohol) is used as a massage for paralysed limbs, cramped limbs, swollen joints, swollen arteries and veins. A brew for the healing of rashes, pimples and sores.

Dose. A Standard brew, using one root finely sliced to three-quarters of a pint of water. Do not heat to boiling point, only slow, gentle heating is permissible for valerian root. Take two tablespoons three times daily before meals. Take more frequently for severe fits, convulsions, etc. Sweeten with honey and add a few drops of an aromatic oil such as oil of peppermint or cloves to disguise the unpleasant taste of valerian.

VERBENA, LEMON-SCENTED (Herb Luisa) (*Lippia citriodora*. Verbenaceae). A cultivated garden shrub, sometimes found wild as a stray. In good soil the shrub can grow quite high, almost into a tree. It is planted beneath verandahs to give shade and to diffuse its almost divine fragrance. It is very typical of Mediterranean gardens (especially the old-fashioned ones) and of the Middle East. It is distinguished by its bright green, narrow leaves, dotted with glands which contain the sweet-smelling, lemon-like oil that gives this herb its special fragrance. Its flowers also have a lemon fragrance and are borne in terminal spikes, in small lacy wands of whitish grey, silver or very pale blue. In Mediterranean countries this herb is called Luisa after Maria Luisa, the royal herbalist whose favourite herb it was. It is also a great favourite of mine and I plant it as close to my door as possible wherever I live long enough to make a garden. In the Canary Islands I was interested to hear that it is so esteemed it is called *La Reina Luisa*, the Queen herb. There it is famed as a remedy for toothache (as I shall describe below) and is often found as a potherb, placed outside windows to waft its sweet fragrance into the home. Its scent can be described as lemon-like, but yet more fragrant than the true lemon tree. Its strong perfume makes it a popular tea-herb, and it is also esteemed as a powerful, non-addictive sedative. In fact, this is a herb very kind to the nerves, and is a general soother, so much so that in the Balearic Isles I found that orthodox vets were prescribing it for curing colic pains in cattle and horses. Its fragrance is utilized in sachets for placing under pillows and in clothes-closets where it also gives some protection against moths. It is popular in babies' cradles, and my children certainly enjoyed the sweet scent.

Use. As a general tonic. As an important nerve remedy as, strangely, it is both a stimulant and a calmative. As a remedy for sleeplessness. To cure nervous spasms. As a soothing tea, especially favoured by infants and the elderly. To soothe aches of the stomach and the intestines. As a remedy for aching teeth and ears. For this purpose a pulp is made of the leaves, preferably fresh not dried, and this is spread on to pads of cotton wool made very hot by being dipped into boiling water and squeezed as dry as possible. The hot herbal pads are then held tightly against the aching teeth or ears. If preferred, the cotton wool can be dipped into hot vegetable oil instead of water.

Dose. Usually taken as a tea in any quantity desired. Pills can also be made of the herb, fresh or dried, finely minced and rolled in thick honey.

VERVAIN (*Verbena officinalis*. Verbenaceae). Found on dry, barren lands. Leaves are spare and opposite, greyish, on square stems. Flowers are small, pale lilac, hooded. Vervain has long been considered as a cure-all, and along with Red Clover is known as God's gift to man. It was a favourite of the great healer Hippocrates, and had even been worshipped by the peasants of Greece, Italy and by the Druids. It is beneficial in all the ills of man, but especially valuable for all fevers, nervous disorders, eye ailments and as a vermifuge. In the plague years, vervain was one of the herbs recommended as a safeguard. An esteemed fertility herb.

Use. Treatment of all infectious ailments and fevers. Treatment of nervous disorders including paralysis and mental stress; excellent for averting convulsions. For liver complaints, gall-stones, weak heart. For pulmonary ailments, including asthma, pneumonia, tuberculosis, whooping-cough. Externally: for weak, sore or inflamed eyes, sore mouths and throats, ulcers of the mouth and gums, and for treatment of all external sores.

Dose. Make a Standard brew and take a wineglass morning and night.

VINE (Wild Grape) (*Vitis vinifera*. Vitaceae). Found on sunny banks and trailing over rocks, also climbing on trees in woodlands, in its natural habitat. Leaves are five-lobed (like cool, green, healing human hands), tender, shining, and of a brilliant green. Flowers are green-yellow, fragrant, gummy. The fruits are the precious grapes, symbol of health and fertility through the ages, a supreme food and medicinal herb. The juice of the fruits of this shrub, taken fresh or fermented into wine, has graced the board since men first gathered around tables to feast and celebrate!

When the human body has become sick almost beyond reasonable hope of recovery, there is still, to my mind, one recourse: for the patient to retire to the neighbourhood of some vineyard where grapes are cultivated by natural methods (that is without artificial fertilizers, chemical sprays, and heavy irrigation), and there to follow a grape cure, living only on the fruit (with a few vine leaves and tendrils also) and drinking only pure water and perhaps fresh goat or sheep milk.

Use. General tonic for the whole system. Treatment of rickets, anaemia, infertility, fevers, impure blood, eczema, lymphatic ailments, dysentery, constipation. Some cases of cancer have been treated with the leaves, vine tendrils, and fruits, but there must be much more evidence and many more trials before one is entitled to make strong claims here. I should like, though, to learn more about this. Externally: as a hair tonic and wound application, use the leaves. Use the juice to dissolve internal growths, especially in uterus and breast.

Dose. As a general tonic eat a few tendrils raw daily. Eat as much of the fruit as desired, during the grape season; chew some of the pips. Take further grapes as fresh juice preserved with honey, and when grapes are out of season, take some wine. Make a Standard brew of the leaves (and a few tendrils), and drink a cup morning and night, sweetened with honey. Use vine tea in a strong brew, as a hair tonic. Leaves of the vine are much used in Greek, Turkish and other *cuisines*.

Stuff vine leaves with boiled rice and white cheese and thin slices of olives, sew up with cotton, and bake lightly until the leaves are soft (a Greek peasant recipe. In the island of Crete the flowers of vegetable marrows are used in the same way as the vine leaves, stuffed with rice, etc.).

The dried fruits — raisins — act both as a laxative and a cure for dysentery. For use as a laxative soak overnight a dozen raisins in a half-cup of water sweetened with one dessertspoon honey. To cure diarrhoea, eat six to eight dry raisins every two hours, during the day. Make the night a long fasting period.

Grape wine is an excellent vehicle for other herbs which may be steeped in it.

VIOLET (Sweet) (*Viola odorata*. Violaceae). Found along shady lane-sides and in woodlands. Leaves are heart-shaped, dark green, flowers viola shaped, deep purple or white — these are very sweetly and strongly perfumed.

The flowers and leaves are mucilaginous and powerfully dissolvent. They have long been used, as many Herbals describe, in internal and external treatment of cancer. The leaves, crushed, are employed as poultices to treat skin cancers and growths. Having emollient properties they are used also for skin lotions and salves. The root is mildly aperient. Violet has a very soothing effect on the head area, taken internally as a tea, applied externally as a cold pack. Violets also provide a delicious sweetmeat. For sugared violets, dip whole flowers in a mixture of melted cane sugar, lemon juice and egg-white. The sugar coating should set hard when dropped into cold water.

Use. Used internally and externally for treatment of tumours, boils, abscesses, pimples, swollen glands and malignant growths, liver and kidney ailments, gall-stones. To calm deranged nerves, improve weak memory, soothe the restless.

Dose. Take a half-dozen leaves or so, raw in the salad; the flowers can also be eaten raw, twice daily with the midday and evening meal. Also a strong tea can be made of the leaves and flowers, two teaspoons of violet to a large cup of water. Externally: apply the leaves raw, binding them over the area to be treated. Or macerate the leaves and flowers and mix them into a base of melted cold cream or vegetable fat, and apply warmed.

VIRGIN'S BOWER (or OLD MAN'S BEARD, or TRAVELLER'S JOY) (*Clematis virginica*. Ranunculaceae). Found as a climbing plant in hedgerows and woodlands. Leaves vine-shaped, bright green turning attractive reds and yellows in the autumn. Flowers are insignificant, pale yellow, producing masses of downy seed material which covers the hedges with grey feathery billows which explain the popular name of 'Old Man's Beard'. Its botanical name indicates its resemblance to a vine — shoots of a vine.

The leaves and flowers are stimulating and tonic. In olden times wayfaring people used to pluck traveller's joy from the hedges and use it as a tea, and as a 'pick-up' when infused in their bottles of ale, also as a headache cure: a head-cloth was soaked in the cold tea and bound over the brow; headaches were inevitable with long hours on the dusty roads in the age of foot or horse-back travel. Externally, the herb was used for treatment of all kinds of sores, including travel blisters on the feet, saddle blisters on buttocks, festering bites from flies, and as a lotion to remove dust from travellers' eyes. The leaves, used as a poultice, had some repute as an external treatment for tumours.

Use. Treatment of all aches and ailments of the wayfarer, from headache and inflamed eyes to blistered and aching feet and bites and stings of insects. Internally, as a tea, externally as a lotion and as a poultice. For the once-prevalent ringworm they used a strong brew mixed with a half-lemon to two table-spoons of the brew.

Dose. A Standard brew of the leaves or flowers or both. A small cupful to be taken to allay pain: sweeten with honey. Externally: steep a cloth in the brew and apply cold. Rinse the eyes with the cold brew. Place fresh leaves of traveller's joy inside the shoes, within the socks, to prevent blisters during long travels on foot.

WATER-CRESS (*Nasturtium officinale*. Cruciferae). Found alongside and within flowing streams of sweet water, also by springs (the love of this plant for pure water fosters the belief that wherever it grows the water is safe to drink: in these days of water pollution, this may no longer be true). Leaves consist of many leaflets, of a brilliant green, and with a biting, tangy taste. Flowers are tiny, white, borne in corymbs. This is an

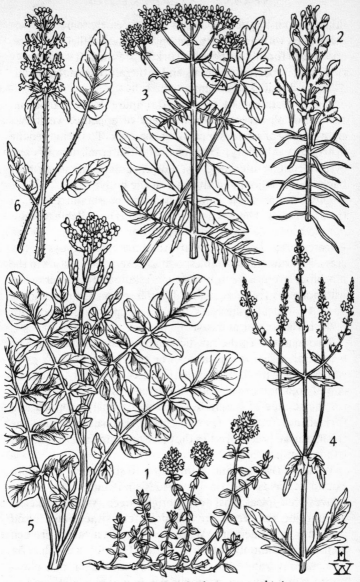

Plate 15. 1. Thyme   2. Toad Flax   3. Valerian
4. Vervain   5. Watercress   6. Wood Betony

important antiseptic herb and is also extremely tonic. It is one more herb with an old reputation for cancer relief and cure, and is used for this purpose by Turkish peasants. It is extremely rich in all important minerals and is therefore in much favour as a blood tonic and anaemia remedy.

Use. Treatment of weak and impure blood, anaemia, rickets, of all nervous ailments, lack of appetite, weak eyesight, failing or scanty supply of breast-milk. To strengthen the heart, cure infertility. Treatment of all internal tumours and cysts including uterine cysts. For rheumatic ailments, stiff back, and stiff joints in any part of the body.

Dose. Eat as much water-cress as can be obtained, raw, in the daily salad. There is no better salad herb available to man. An old name for water-cress was 'Poor-man's bread'. When wheaten bread could not be afforded there was always watercress. The raw seeds, a tablespoon as dose, taken fasting in the morning, are a cure for worm infestation. In winter when water-cress is freely available it is the season for making the good Provençal watercress soup. The cress is cooked with milk, garlic, butter and cayenne pepper.

Two handfuls of the raw herb eaten daily cannot fail to be beneficial; larger quantities can be taken if desired. A good way of taking this biting hot herb is to chop it finely, steep in a cup of cold milk, then drink the water-cress-infused milk and eat the residue of the herb. Can also be finely chopped and forked into fresh, soft white cheese. Externally: apply the fresh, crushed herb direct to the place requiring treatment, and bandage in position.

WHEAT (*Triticum* and *Agropyrum* — species. Gramineae). Found in fields and on bank-sides and under cultivation. Leaves are typical grass-form, bright green, shiny. Spikelets are upright, the grains are rounded, fat, without awns, and turn dark gold when ripe. Wheat is one of the most nutritive of all plants, commonly known as 'the staff of life'. It is rich in fat and carbohydrates and some protein, and has a high phosphorous and iron content and is rich in vitamins A, B, and E. The germ (heart) of wheat is now proved a vital food and medicine for the human body and an important nerve tonic. The bran (outer skin of the grains) is also highly medicinal and has external as well as internal use.

Use. As a nutritive food and tonic for all parts of the body; an important brain food. The germ can be taken raw as a digestive and nerve tonic, anaemia remedy and rickets cure. The bran as a nerve tonic, constipation, gentle laxative.

Dose. Wheat can be eaten raw, merely sprinkle on to a shallow dish of the grains enough cold water to cover them. Leave in a sunny (or warm) place until germination — i.e. until grains sprout — usually 2-3 days. Then eat raw, or crushed, mixed with flour, and formed into small, flat, cakes, and lightly baked. Wholewheat flour, as bread, is the true 'staff of life'. Add raw bran to soups. Take it raw, several teaspoons with other meals, to cure constipation. Use bran as a poultice. Fill a tub with hot water, stir in a half-pound of bran, and give a bran bath for curing skin ailments.

WHITE POND LILY (WHITE LILY) (*Nymphaea alba*. Nymphaeaceae). Found on ponds, lakes and other still waters; leaves are very large and round, dark green, and float flat on the surface of the water. Flowers are beautiful, large, solitary, rounded of form, sweetly scented and with prominent yellow stamens. The name is from the Greek for water-nymph, as this lily has the paleness of the nymphs and like them inhabits the waters. The root is the part used, and it is very soothing, cooling and astringent, also possesses antiseptic properties. The leaves are sometimes used for binding over wounds or inflamed areas of the skin. The Yellow Pond Lily (*Nuphar lutea*. Nymphaeaceae), is also medicinal. Extolled by the great herbalist of ancient times, Dioscorides. Has also the common name of 'Brandy-bottle', from the brandy-like scent of its flowers and the shape of its seed-vessels, which are like the traditional brandy-flagons. Leaves of *Nuphar lutea* have healing virtues similar to those of *Nymphaea alba*.

Use. Treatment of diarrhoea, and all bowel ailments, leucorrhoea (internally and externally). Expels excess mucus from all parts of the body and reduces internal inflammations. Good in dropsy and for kidney disorders. For soothing the bowels: very helpful for infants in this respect. It has given relief when other herbal treatments have failed. Externally: as a vaginal douche. As a gargle for throat ailments and as a wash for sore mouths and gums. As a nasal douche for congestion of the nose and nasal passages. The leaves are used externally for treatments of all kinds of inflammations of the skin and genital organs, and for cure of wounds, sores, rashes and sunburn.

Dose. Take a piece of root about six inches long, shave into fine pieces, and place in a half-pint of cold water. Heat gently for five minutes, keeping below boiling point. Steep for at least three hours, strain and use. Take a tablespoon morning and night, more often in bowel ailments. Externally: use the same brew, as a douche, gargle, lotion and skin application. Use the leaves raw, straight from the water.

WINTERGREEN (*Pyrola secunda*. Pyrolaceae). Found in woodlands, particularly fir-tree woods. A rather shrubby plant. Leaves are oval with serrated edges. Flowers are small and greenish white and quite fragrant. They are borne in racemes and are peculiar in all leaning one way. This herb takes its name from the word for a pear tree, as there is supposed to be a resemblance to pear-blossom. The American species is the 'Chimaphila' of the North American Indians, and a greatly treasured herb in their herbal-lore. The whole plant is a powerful diuretic, used in all ailments of the bladder and kidneys. Externally it is one more useful poultice herb. There is another American herb known as Wintergreen; this is *Gaultheria procumbens* which produces the well-known and edible berry called bear-berry or partridge berry avidly sought out by the named creatures. *Betula lenta* (Sweet Birch) yields a 'Wintergreen oil' used against sciatica.

Use. Treatment of all inflammations and obstructions of the bladder and kidneys. Also for dropsy and rheumatism. Externally, as a poultice in treatment of boils and ulcers. A solution of the leaves provides a good gargle for infections of the mouth and throat. The extracted oil of Wintergreen, mixed with vinegar, preferably apple vinegar, is a good rub for rheumatic inflammations and swellings, arthritis, stiff or swollen joints, stiff back, muscular pains and all kinds of sprains.

Dose. Make a tea of the leaves alone or the leaves and flowers, and take two dessertspoons night and morning. As a poultice merely warm the leaves over hot steam, pulp up and apply where needed. As a gargle and mouth-wash, soak the leaves in cider vinegar for twenty-four hours, then dilute the solution with two parts of water to every one of vinegar, and use warm. An old-fashioned remedy for sore throats and stiff necks, which is very effective, is to soak sheets of brown paper in the wintergreen-apple vinegar solutions and then bandage the prepared paper around the neck. Wear this all night. Two layers of treated paper are generally used. If you use oil of Wintergreen, mix one part of oil to six of vinegar, and add one part of cayenne pepper to every part of oil.

WITCH HAZEL (*Hamamelis virginiana.* Hamamelidaceae). Found in woodlands and by water-sides. Leaves resemble the common hazel shrub, but are smaller and have deeper veining. Its flowers are spectacular, being bright yellow with petals of slender spidery form, forming delicate corollas like incurved chrysanthemums. This is one of the sacred herbs of the American Indians who claim magical healing powers for this beautiful shrub. It is both refrigerant and astringent, one of the supreme wound herbs. Difficult to prepare in the home, it is available as an extract in pharmacies. Extract of witch hazel is very popular as a skin tonic and as an application for bruises.

Use. Internally and externally to check haemorrhages from all parts of the body, including nose bleeding, bleeding from the womb, bleeding after tooth extraction. Also used to check milk leakage from the breasts. For treatment of internal ulcers of the stomach and intestines, for healing internal burns resulting from intake of poisons such as phosphorus, sulphuric acid. More drastic methods will of course precede this healing process. Externally as a douche for treatment of leucorrhoea, vaginitis. Apply extract of witch hazel direct to burns, scalds, cuts, bruises, sore breasts, sore eyes (use in dilution) and for bed sores and blisters, foot blisters, and piles. As a gargle for sore and inflamed throats, and for ulcerated gums and throats.

Dose. A teaspoonful in a half-wineglass of warm water. Or it may be taken on lumps of sugar. Externally: apply extract of witch hazel neat. For a douche, two teaspoons of witch hazel extract to a pint of tepid water. For a gargle, a half-teaspoon to a cup of water. To check nose bleeding, sniff similar dilution (as for gargle) up the nostrils and retain this for as long as possible. If necessary use double strength. For deep wounds apply on swabs of sphagnum moss or cotton wool.

WOOD BETONY (*Betonica officinalis*. Labiatae). Found in woods and under dense hedges. Leaves are sparse, serrated, rough, dark. Flowers are tubular, lipped, dark. This rather hairy plant grows several feet high. Its botanical names come from the Celtic, from *ben* a word for head, and *ton*, meaning good or tonic. This valuable herb does possess most powerful influence over the head region and is therefore a true cephalic. It is much used in the treatment of headache and neuralgia of the head and face, and will relieve most pains of this nature. As it opens up congested areas of the liver and spleen, it is a valued remedy for jaundice.

Use. Treatment of all nervous ailments, convulsions, hysterical delirium, fainting. It will also soothe the stomach, cure biliousness and expel worms. Externally, it will cure bites and stings of all types of insects and animals, including the poisonous ones.

Dose. A Standard brew of the leaves. Take a wineglass morning and night. Can also be brewed in port wine, a tablespoon of the herb to a pint bottle. Dose, the same.

WOODRUFF (*Asperula odorata*. Rubiaceae). Found in woodlands. Leaves are tiny, dark and in whorls. Flowers are in terminal corymbs, and are tiny, white, frail and most sweetly scented. The whole herb is aromatic, and the scent even increases on drying, and this is exploited by putting bunches of woodruff in linen closets and similar places. It is a tonic and nervine herb, and despite its tiny size it increases the flow of breast milk. It is one of the 'tea' herbs of the English gypsies.

Use. Treatment of nervous debility, poor memory, depression, hysteria, frigidity. Also for jaundice, chronic constipation, acid stomach. For all fevers, excellent in childbirth fever. To produce easy flow of milk in women and milch animals. Externally for wounds and ringworm, and as a rub to strengthen wasted limbs.

Dose. A handful of the whole herb infused in wine for several days. Take two tablespoons three times daily before meals. For fevers make a Standard brew and drink a small cupful night and morning, more often in childbirth fever. Externally: use the Standard brew as a lotion, except for ringworm, when the herb should be infused in light beer for several days, and the lotion then applied three times daily. As a rub, infuse the oil, a handful of herb to a pint bottle of oil. (*See* Herbal Oils.)

WOOD SAGE (*Teucrium scorodonia*. Labiatae). Found in shady places. Likes hedgerows and woodlands. Leaves are rough, downy, rather dark and have a slight garlic odour (one of its common names being 'Garlic sage'). Flowers are in spikes, and are greenish yellow and hooded. In addition to garlic scent the plant also has an aroma of hops. It is a very bitter-tasting herb. Wood sage has been used from ancient times as a blood-cleansing tea. It also shares with garlic the claim to be the most effective mucus expellent, and has some reputation as a cancer herb, especially when the cancer is external, and wood sage is employed as a poultice. Treatment of fevers, colds, blood disorders and breast ailments, especially mastitis.

Use. For coughs, colds, blood disorders and breast ailments, including mastitis. Also for pneumonia, bronchitis, general catarrh. Internal tumours, and obstructions, boils, rheumatism, gout. Externally as a poultice for all skin ailments, tumours, mastitis, boils, styes, skin cancer.

Dose. Standard brew, two tablespoons three times a day. Sweeten with honey. Use the Standard brew, unsweetened, as a lotion. For a poultice, use the entire herb.

WOOD SORREL (*Oxalis acetosella*. Oxalidaceae). The only British member of the large family. Found in woodlands and on shady banksides. Leaves are of shamrock form, pale green, frail, and have purple undersides. Flowers are bell shaped, silvery-white with green or purple veining, and are solitary and very frail. The strong oxalic acid content of this delicate plant gives it its generic name meaning 'acid' or 'sharp'. Its powerful medicinal properties are belied by its delicate form. It is powerfully antiseptic and refrigerant, useful therefore in fevers and the cleansing of an impure blood-stream. It increases flow of urine, and this power, combined with its other medicinal virtues, makes it an ideal herb for treatment of ailments of the kidneys and bladder. Externally it is used for eye treatments, and to cool and soothe rashes and inflamed areas in any part of the body, and for the healing of scrofulous ulcers. The expressed juice is also a treatment for unsightly freckles when they have become too numerous to be attractive. One peasant method of preparing sorrel leaves for external use, is to wrap a handful of the herb in a cabbage leaf and to macerate it in warm ashes until all is reduced to a pulp. Wood Sorrel is a favourite of the American Indians. They used to feed the pulped roots to their horses to increase their speed, 'to put the North Wind into their hooves'. This might be a tip for athletes, for the roots of wood sorrel are edible for humans also. A small vase of the flowers placed in a sick room is said to keep it fresh and make the atmosphere cooler.

It is claimed for wood sorrel that this is the original Seamrog or Shamrock of Ireland, a plant to which magic properties are attributed. However, the Dutch Clover has taken over the name of 'Shamrock' nowadays.

There is another form of *Oxalis* with similar leaves, but without the purple shading, and with long-stemmed flowers, not solitary, three or more on a stem of a yellow colour. This sorrel has similar medicinal virtues to *acetosella* except for not being quite so blood-cooling.

Use. Treatment of all fevers, especially those producing a hot rash or pimples. Treatment of impure blood, high blood-

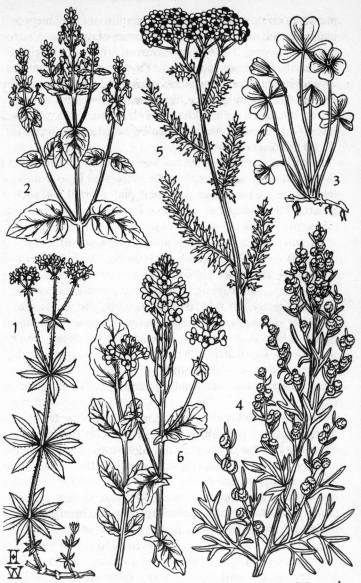

Plate 16. 1. Woodruff 2. Wood Sage 3. Wood Sorrel
4. Wormwood 5. Yarrow 6. Yellow Rocket

pressure, varicose veins. For inflammation of the kidneys and bladder, acid, urine, vaginitis, hot flushes of the face. Also for mentstrual irregularities, diseases of the sexual glands. Externally for treatment of all skin rashes, inflammations, wounds, burns, scalds, varicose veins (bind leaves around the legs at night, held in place by cabbage leaves with an upper cotton bandage); for freckles (apply a lotion of the expressed juice — some cucumber juice can be added with advantage); for all minor eye ailments.

Dose. Eat a handful of the raw leaves once daily, a few of the flowers as well. Sorrel can also be macerated in sour milk, a tablespoon of the leaves to a half-pint of milk; it adds a pleasant sour taste to the milk and imparts to it its medicinal properties. Drink a cupful twice daily before meals.

External use: a Standard lotion can be made of the leaves and/or flowers. Or the leaves can be bruised and steeped in oil for several days. (*See* Herbal oils.) For eye ailments use the lotion only. The leaves can also be crushed to a pulp and applied directly, for skin treatments, burns and scalds, etc.

WORMWOOD (*Artemisia absinthium*. Compósitae). Found on waste land in dry regions, sometimes in the desert, also on rocky land. Cultivated in herb gardens. Leaves are greyish, fringed, and covered with short silken down. Flowers are in erect panicles, and are small, greenish-yellow, globular in form.

The whole plant is extremely aromatic and bitter tasting, its bitterness being mentioned in the Bible. This pungency and bitterness are due to the presence of absinthate of potassium and a quantity of green camphorated volatile oil. It yields what the druggists call *absinthe*. This bitter principle is used to make the tonic wine of France, Absinthe. Over-use of this potent wine was found to cause epilepsy, and brought into ill repute a herb so beneficial that the Greek goddess Artemis chose this plant for her own. She received such health benefits from wormwood that she gave it her own name in place of the former one of 'parthensis'. Many other herbs have been harmed by misuse of extracts derived from them. In antiquity wormwood was chosen as a symbol of health, and healers painted it on their doors as a sign to their patients. I would happily paint wormwood on my door, for it is one of my chosen herbs and I make great use of it in my herbal work. The Provence peasants say of wormwood that if women realized the good that it could do them, they would wear it around their heads as a crown to do honour to this remarkable herb. The great healer Saint John the Baptist, habitually wore a girdle woven from wormwood, and one of the common names is 'St. John's Girdle'. Its medicinal properties are primarily antiseptic, nervine, vermifuge and narcotic. Like all 'bitters' it is a good tonic and aid to digestion. Externally it is an insecticide and general antiseptic.

Use. Treatment of all fevers, infestations by worms, enteritis, constipation, jaundice. To restore appetite, allay pains from indigestion, stimulate deficient gastric juices, cure diarrhoea and dysentery. For all women's ailments, including leucorrhoea, morning sickness, threatened miscarriage. Also obesity, dropsy, constipation. Externally and internally to check undue falling of hair and baldness. To cleanse the human body of vermin, such as lice and fleas. Combined with other herbs as a repellent for stinging or biting insects or animals, and to soothe bites of such a nature. As a treatment for ear troubles and to soothe earache.

Dose. Wormwood is a potent herb (its over-use will increase unduly the action of the heart and the blood-vessels). It should not be taken for over-long periods in over-large doses. In proper dosage, a long-esteemed herb to safeguard and strengthen the human body, especially the female body. Make a Standard brew, weak, using only three sprigs of wormwood cut to about six inches in length, to a pint of water, and take two tablespoons morning and night during the prescribed period of treatment, which is usually until the symptoms vanish, when the use of wormwood should be discontinued. Sweeten with honey to disguise the bitterness of this herb.

YARROW (*Achillea millefolium*. Compositae). Found along waysides and in pastures. Leaves are greyish, finely feathered and pungent. Flowers are in corymbs of white or pink disk-form flowers. The whole plant has a biting and bitterish taste which is not unpleasant. Indeed sheep and goats seek it out for its tonic properties and peppery taste. This is a herb long known for its powers in the healing of wounds. The Greek warrior and athlete Achilles gave this herb its name. It is told that he was the first to discover its medicinal virtues, and that by using yarrow blossoms he healed his own battle wounds and those of his soldiers.

The peculiar fragrance and taste of yarrow are due to the presence of achilleic and tannic acids, also an essential oil of yarrow and a bitter extractive. The plant will yield its properties to water or alcohol. Apart from its use in the treatment of wounds and all types of haemorrhages it is also a great fever herb owing to its peculiar power of dilating the skin pores and producing copious sweating. It is often used by peasants as a substitute for quinine, and is quite as effective and far safer than that drug. Sometimes used for beer in place of hops.

Use. Treatment of all fevers, including intermittent fevers. It is much used in smallpox and typhoid fever as well as for malaria. For colds, headache, diarrhoea, dysentery: for diarrhoea of infants. Its astringent properties are effective for checking haemorrhage and over-profuse menstruation.

Also for pneumonia, pleurisy, inflamed throat, rheumatism. For hysteria, epilepsy, trembling. Externally: all wounds, ulcers old and new, fistulas, soft tumours. To check falling of the hair (bathe the head with yarrow brew and massage also with salve made from the flowers): to quell toothache, chew the leaves; for earache apply some of the lotion quite hot to the ears, and insert a few drops of cooler lotion. Use as a douche in diarrhoea, dysentery (as well as taking as an internal medicine), also for piles and womb troubles. In oil infusion to repel mosquitoes.

Dose. Make a Standard brew. Take a wineglass morning and night, sweetened with honey. For external use make a stronger brew, doubling the amount of herb to the same given amount of water. In fevers give the patient a yarrow bath, tossing several handfuls of yarrow into a bath of hot water, as well as giving drinks of yarrow brew. To make a salve of the flowers, melt cold cream or vegetable fat and work into this the finely cut blossoms; add a little bees-wax if possible, to help the salve to solidify. In earache, in addition to use of the warm yarrow lotion, a wad of the crushed leaves, well warmed, can be placed in each ear.

YELLOW ROCKET (Winter-cress) (*Barbarea vulgaris*. Cruciferae). Found in hedgerows, pasture land and in gardens. Leaves are small and pinnate. Flowers are small, yellow, crossform and shedding their petals readily. Seed pods are prominent, long and narrow, four angled. The plant grows from one to two feet high, and has a stout and glabrous stem. It is found in winter-time. It is dedicated to Saint Barbara, who blessed it: hence its generic name. This is a peppery, biting herb, antiseptic, healing, tonic and cheering to the human spirit. The Arabs use it in milk to safeguard health when their herds are not in the best of condition.

Use. Treatment of colds, catarrh, indigestion, stomach disorders, flatulence, lack of appetite. As a general tonic, to give internal warmth in winter weather, and to banish depression. As a vermifuge and rheumatism remedy.

Dose. The seed pods: Eat six or so raw pods morning and night. For treatment of worms, double this dose.

4

Recipes (Cosmetic, Medicinal, Culinary and Other)

All who work with herbs have many recipes, which they have gathered together over the years. Here, I am giving around fifty, ranging from the recipes which are of culinary use at home, utilizing herbs (including cereals and fruits), to toilet preparations, beverages and medicines. In the preceding chapter of Materia Medica, there are recipes included in the text.

In this chapter several recipes include leaves of trees not featured in this book, but such leaves can be obtained easily and the recipes are favourites of mine, so I have used them.

TOILET PREPARATIONS

Tooth-powder. Make a vegetable charcoal by burning slices of bread to charcoal. Pound the black slices into a fine powder. Flavour with a few drops of oil of peppermint or of clove or rosemary. Brush the teeth with this, morning and night, using a soft brush and cold water.

Tooth-powder (*stain remover*). Sage leaves and common sea salt, rubbed well together, then baked until hard. Pound into a fine powder. Rub the teeth with this every morning and evening. This will take away all yellow film and stains. (Many Swiss peasants and Bedouin Arabs clean their teeth merely by rubbing with sage leaves.) Try the juice of fresh strawberries on cotton wool brushed over the teeth to give shining whiteness.

Tooth-paste (Vanilla tooth-paste—French). Vegetable charcoal powdered, one ounce, white honey (clover will do) one ounce, vanilla sugar one ounce, Peruvian bark (quinine bark) a half ounce, and a few drops of any essential oil, such as peppermint, or drops of tincture of lavender. The vanilla sugar can be made by triturating (rubbing to a powder) a teaspoon of saturated tincture of vanilla with an ounce of icing sugar, and drying the mixture by employing a gentle heat. Mix the powdered ingredients together, then blend into the honey and the flavourings. Press into a glass pot and use on a damp toothbrush.

Cleansing Cream (for the face and hands). Oil of sweet almonds three ounces, white wax half an ounce, lanolin one ounce, rose-water one ounce, oil of jasmine ten drops, oil of rose geranium ten drops (or other flower oils can be used, such as lavender, rosemary, orange blossom). Beat together the white wax and lanolin in a double boiler. Beat hard again, adding almond oil. Slowly blend in the rose-water. Remove from heat, and when new-milk-warm add the floral oils, drop by drop. Pour into jars to set. Do not use plastic containers.

Complexion Lotion (Elder Blossom). Heat slowly a handful of elder blossoms in a half-pint of buttermilk or cheese whey. Do not heat above warm — new-milk-warm. Keep on heat for thirty minutes or so, until the blossom softens. Remove from heat and allow to steep for three hours. Reheat and add an ounce of white honey. Use cold, to apply to face, neck and hands. Cools, softens and cleanses the skin.

Eye Lotion (Cucumber). From a six-inch slice of fresh cucumber squeeze the juice. Add two tablespoons of whey to this, and apply to the eyes, internally and externally. If whey is not available, the cucumber juice can be used neat. Cools and soothes inflamed eyes, tones up the membranes of the eyes.

Hair Tonic and Setting Lotion. Cut up a handful of sage leaves and tops and the same quantity of rosemary. Place in a pint of cold water and bring slowly to the boil. Simmer for three minutes (keep covered throughout). Remove from heat and allow to steep for three hours. Do not strain, merely pour off the required quantity for massaging into the scalp and hair every night. The lotion is improved by adding ten drops of oil of rosemary; or natural eau-de-cologne (not synthetic), can be added. Tones the hair, sets the hair, improves its colour, removes scurf. (For darkening, add Indian tea.)

Hair-growing Oil (Willow and Maidenhair fern). Take a handful each of willow leaves and maidenhair fern and heat them slowly in a half-pint of salad oil into which three cloves have been tossed. Heat gently, by standing the container in hot water over a low flame. Keep on the heat for one hour. Do not strain until cold. Then strain and pour into glass jars or clay crocks. Massage the scalp with the herbal oil every night.

Spirits of Lavender (Tonic lotion). A few drops also can be taken internally on loaf sugar for nervous ailments and mental depression. Dried lavender flowers, two tablespoons, one grated nutmeg, two teaspoonfuls of cinnamon, sweet cecily leaves (if available) one tablespoon. Pulverize all the ingredients and mix well together. Add a quart of pure alcohol. Let the mixture stand and steep in a warm place (sunlight is good), and shake well once daily. Then strain off and bottle, capping tightly. Excellent applied on cloths wrung out in cold water, and placed over the forehead, to allay headache, soothe fevers. In fevers also apply to the pulse on the wrists.

Queen of Hungary's Water. Follow the same recipe as for spirits of lavender, but using tops and flowers of fresh rosemary instead of the dried lavender, using double the amount, and omit the sweet cecily leaves. Similar use to spirits of lavender.

Pot Pourri (Provence). Gather as many as possible of the following kinds of scented flowers: petals of the pale red and dark red roses, moss roses and damask roses, also acacia, and the heads of pinks, violets, lily of the valley, lilacs — of blue and white — orange blossom and lemon blossom, mignonette, heliotrope, narcissi and jonquils: with a *small* proportion of the flowers of balm, rosemary, thyme and myrtle. Spread them out to dry, and as they become fully dry in turn, put them into a tall glass jar, with alternate layers of coarse salt, mixed with powdered orris root (use two parts of salt to one of orris). Pack the flowers and salt-orris, until the vessel is filled. Close the jar for one month, then stir all up and moisten with sufficient rose-water to penetrate to the lowest layer. Cap with a muslin cloth tightly tied, and use in cotton bags to scent linen closets, etc. Used also for scenting writing-paper (in former days!).

Scented Powder (1) (*Poudre à la Mareschale*). Take one pound of moss scraped from oak trees (a grey moss, called 'lungs of oak' by the American Indians and used for treatment of wounds), found commonly on oak trees. Reduce the moss to a powder, after well drying it. Add a half-pound of common starch. Take also, all reduced to powder, of calamus root one ounce, cyperus, one ounce, rotten oak-wood powder, one ounce, cloves a half-ounce. Mix well. Cyperus is a perennial, rush-like plant related to papyrus and mariscus.

(2) (*Poudre d'acacia*). Take one pound of powdered orris root, half a pound of dried and powdered acacia flowers, two ounces dried bergamot peel, quarter ounce of powdered cloves, and several heads of the sweet-scented purple-flowered wild orchis, *Gymnadenia conopsea*. Pound all together. The bergamot orange is much like the Seville, but pear-shaped, and its acid pulp is very fragrant.

(3) (*Poudre de Chypre*). Oak-moss is macerated in water (preferably spring water — bottled Vichy water, etc., can be used). Steep the moss in the water for several days, and then submit it to strong pressure in a cotton cloth. Then moisten with rose-water mixed with one-third of orange-flower water. Soak the oak moss, adding rose and orange-flower water until the moss has absorbed to full capacity. Then press the moss further and pulverize it. This *poudre de Chypre* is used as a basis for other flower perfumes, and greatly increases their powers.

Lotion for a Fragrant Breath. Take half a pint of sherry wine and into this put an ounce each of powdered cloves, grated nutmeg and a half-ounce each of ground cinnamon and bruised caraway seeds. Place all in a pint flask and allow to stand for three days, shaking the mixture well morning and night. Finely strain the mixture through a cheese-cloth and add ten drops of spirits of lavender (*see* earlier recipe). A few drops of this wine mixture taken on loaf sugar, will give a fragrant breath. A few drops can be added to water to make an excellent gargle.

REMEDIES

A Gargle. Take a handful each of elder blossom and sage leaves and tops, and make a brew in a half-pint of cold water. Add a heaped teaspoon of honey, a half-teaspoon of oil of sweet almonds, and five drops of oil of cloves. Gargle with this frequently to ease a sore throat and to allay a cough.

A Throat Pack. Soak a piece of linen or cotton cloth in castor oil, to which has been added six drops of camphorated oil to every four ounces of castor oil. (Do not use woollen cloth.) Place on an enamel or tin plate in the oven and heat until the linen begins to singe. Apply the cloth to the throat when as hot as can just be tolerated, wrapping well around the whole area. Then bind into place with a broad cotton bandage, and wear this all night. Effective for treatment of sore throat or stiff neck; also for swollen glands and mumps.

Remedy for a Cold. Soften a handful of rosemary tops in warm water, then plunge them into a pint of hot cider. Add a pinch of ground cayenne pepper and a pinch of ground ginger; drink hot. Alternate with strong tea of sage and borage with honey.

Remedy for colds and fevers. Wash a medium-size juicy lemon. Cut it through with six cuts, but do not remove the skin. Place the lemon, point downwards, in a shallow dish of pure liquid honey in which two cloves are standing, and soak over-night. Then squeeze the lemon dry and take the lemon-honey in teaspoonful doses when required. The natural citric acid thus extracted from the soaked peel is an excellent cure for all kinds of fevers and colds. Can be mixed with a wineglass of warm water if desired.

RECIPES (COSMETIC, MEDICINAL, CULINARY AND OTHER)

A Remedy for earache. Cut up finely a handful of hore-hound. Place in half a pint of cold water, heat, then remove before boiling-point is reached. Steep for four hours. Strain. Add two drops of clove oil to every teaspoon of horehound brew. Drop a teaspoonful into the ears, using at tepid heat. When ear pains are very acute, mix six poppy heads in with the horehound, when the water containing the horehound has become warm.

A Remedy for Weak Eyes. Take some of the young, moist buds of white poplar tree before they open. Fill with warmed honey and press over the eyes, holding them there for five minutes if possible. Strengthens all the eye tissues.

A Chest Rub. Take a handful of the grey lichen (oak moss) from oak trees (*see* recipe *Poudre de Chypre*, already given), and make a strong brew, heating this in a pint of hot ale. Add a few drops of camphorated oil, six drops to the pint, and apply hot to the chest and around the back, in the chest region. Keep the body warm.

A Chilblain Ointment. Take a handful of primrose leaves, steam them gently and then pound them into melted lanolin, until all is absorbed. Add a teaspoon or more of thick honey and work this into the primrose-lanolin. A few drops of oil of thyme can also be added with advantage. Apply the ointment warm to the chilblains and cover the feet with large-size, loose-fitting cotton socks (do not used wool or nylon for this purpose). (A good companion remedy is to persuade the patient to walk barefoot in snow.)

A Toothache Remedy. Soak whole cloves in hot honey, and let the patient chew them slowly, rolling them around the aching tooth. (A well-proved French gypsy remedy.) Nut-galls found in dyer's oak or by *Quercus infectoria*, rich in tannin, were also so used.

A Remedy for Stomach-ache. Take a small handful each of endive and fresh mint and steep them in a pint of white wine for a whole day. Add a teaspoon each of powdered cinnamon and wild thyme and a generous pinch of dill seeds. Strain after steeping and take a wineglass three times daily before meals.

(With severe stomach pains the patient should be fasting on herbal teas only.)

A Remedy for Festering Sores or Whitlows. Heat a whole lemon, make a tunnel down the centre; pack this with common salt and fresh pine needles and place the affected finger within, keeping it buried in the lemon as long as possible. Repeat the treatment as needed until the ailment is cured.

A Rubbing Lotion. Steep a heaped tablespoon of powdered seaweed and one teaspoon of cayenne pepper in hot apple vinegar, add six drops of oil of pine, and use as a rub for stiff and aching joints and other parts of the body where there is stiffness or pain.

Burns and Scalds. Apply slices of raw potato immediately, squeezing the juice on to the burnt or scalded parts. Then apply thick honey to exclude all air. Preferably grate the potato finely.

Another remedy — said to have been handed down by the Crusaders as a relief against burns from oil, when men poured boiling oil down upon their enemies during warfare — warm sweet chestnut leaves in hot water to soften them, place in the air to cool, and when cold lay the wet leaves over the burns. Then cover with a cotton cloth and pour cold tea over the cloth at intervals to keep the cloth cool and moist. This will extract the 'fire' from the burn and prevent scar tissue. The 'tea' part of this recipe was a later refinement, for tea was not drunk in Europe until the seventeenth century. Or 'tea' may have indicated any bland herbal brew.

I have proved instant pain relief in severe burns by gently pressing over the burns the inner (slimey) sides of the peels of ripe bananas, and further binding peels over the area or areas (inner side touching the burn). Change the peels every few hours.

A Worm Remedy. Give a handful of green walnut leaves boiled in milk. About three or four leaves, taken fasting in the early morning for three days or more, until the case is cured.

A 'Green' Surgical Dressing. If people would apply the drawing, cooling, healing and antiseptic powers of the many 'wound' herbs, to wounds from surgery and otherwise, to sores of all kinds, they would in many cases obtain such speedy relief from pain, and in some cases achieve such speedy healing, that they would never again use chemical applications. Throughout the text of Materia Medica chapter, wound herbs are given. The following are the ones which I use most in my herbal work: the tender leaves of cabbage, kale, lettuce, geranium, violet, vine, bind-weed (especially the large leaves of Morning Glory), castor-oil leaves, and those of the water-lily. Use one kind, or a blend of several. Wash the leaves free of dust, snip off all stalks, break down any ridgy veins by pressure, and lay over the wounds, sores, etc. When the leaves heat up from the inflammation and impurities that they have extracted, replace with fresh ones. Bind with damp cotton cloths.

Remedies for Stings. The basis for successful treatment of stings is immediate action. Do not let stings and bites from insects and animals stay untreated, to inflame and swell.

Ants. Pulp up some cloves of garlic or take slices of raw onion and apply at once. Further soothe the irritated parts with cucumber juice or pulped parsley or garlic in vinegar.

Bees and wasps. First remove the sting, then press out the poison from the skin. Soothe the fire of the sting with a paste of whitewash. After an hour wash off as whitewash itself lightly burns the skin. Then soothe with herbal oil, and bind over with leaves of dock or plantain. Or apply the parsley or garlic in vinegar (*see Ants.*)

Scorpions, poisonous spiders, medusa (jelly-fish). If first-aid is necessary, cut the place with the point of a sharp knife and press or suck out (of course, not swallowing) all the surface poison. Then apply the pulped leaves of wormwood, rue and sage, as available. Preferably heat the leaves for a few minutes in hot water to make their volatile oils more easily available to the human skin. Bind in place with cotton bandages soaked in a mixture of hot water and vinegar, equal parts. Even more effective is an application of extracted oils of wormwood, rue and rosemary (see pages 24 and 25), if available: likewise covering with bandages soaked in hot vinegar-water. (I have cured numerous cases of severe bites, several being from the giant species of scorpion, considered fatal, using this treatment.) The most effective and the speediest remedies are the essential oils of these herbs applied on swabs of cotton wool first dampened in hot water.

To keep away mosquitoes and midges when spending evenings out-of-doors. Gather some of the aromatic herbs, such as sage, southernwood rue, rosemary, elecampane and others, add some dry paper or dry grass, place in quite large open cans, sprinkle the herbs, etc. with paraffin and ignite: the pungent smoke will clear the air of mosquitoes and kindred biting insects. The Mexican Indians burn thuja pine.

BEVERAGES

Gorse Blossom Champagne. Take a half-gallon measure of gorse blossoms, one gallon of hot water, one lemon, two pounds cane sugar — (or one and a half pounds sugar and half-pound pure honey) one pound raisins (the large ones if possible), one thick slice of toasted brown bread, and one ounce yeast.

Put blossoms, sugar and hot water into a large enamel bowl and leave for one week. At the end of this period, press down the blossoms and stir well. Do this each day for a week, and then strain out the solids.

Into the strained liquid put the raisins cut small and the lemon thinly sliced. Now spread the slice of bread on both sides with the yeast, and put this to float on the brew. Leave for fourteen days, then skim off any floating residue, and strain further until the liquid is clear and now bottle. *N.B.* The blossoms must be dry for gathering. Be sure to cork the bottles tightly, and use natural cork stoppers, not plastic ones.

(This is a New Forest, England recipe. It was Augustus John, the famous painter, who named this wine 'gorse champagne'. I used to take him bottles of this gorse drink.)

Sunflower Cordial. Take two large handfuls of sunflower seeds and place in a pan. Add one and a half pints of cold water, a slice of lemon (about a finger thick), and a piece of ginger root about four inches long. Bring to just below boiling point and simmer gently until the seeds are soft (approximately one hour or less). Allow to stand and steep. When the cordial is medium-warm, strain it and stir in a small half-cupful of pure honey. Drink cold. (The children can eat up the boiled seeds, extracting their kernels.) (This is a very old recipe, in fact, several hundred years old, from French Canada. Maple syrup was often used to sweeten this healthful delicious beverage.)

Treacle Ginger-beer. Take one pound brown sugar, one ounce bruised ginger root, a quarter ounce hops, and a pinch of saffron. Pour over these ingredients three quarts of water. Boil for a few minutes in the water, strain and add five quarts of cold water. Finally add a tablespoon of fresh yeast. Let the mixture work all night and bottle the following morning, not corking too tightly for several days. Do not fill the bottles to the top, leave several inches for expansion. (A good blood and nerve tonic.)

Kingcup. Pour two pints of hot water on to the outer rind of two well-ripened lemons, two small slices of orange peel and six slices of cucumber. Then add twelve lumps of cane sugar. When cold add leaves of basil, and mint, and sprinkle with powdered cinnamon to taste. (A Provence drink. Honeycomb is often used in place of the sugar, about half a comb.)

Barley Water. Whole barley four ounces, honey two ounces, peel of half a small lemon (well washed), a pint of water. First boil the barley in a little water and throw this away. Then pour the pint of water over the cleaned barley, and add the lemon peel. Simmer gently until the barley is soft. Remove from heat, allow to seep, and add the honey when the barley water is new-milk-warm. (There are many ways of making barley water: this is an old-fashioned recipe and a good-tasting one.)

Oatmeal Gruel. Take two ounces of sweet oatmeal, and mix into a thin paste by gradually adding cold water. Then add salt to taste. Heat a half-pint of cold water and add to this a wineglass of a day-old milk. Before it boils add the oatmeal mixture. Simmer gently but keep well below boiling point.

Cook for three to five minutes. The taste is improved by adding a few sprigs of fragrant herbs such as marjoram or thyme.

Linseed 'Tea'. Soak overnight two ounces of linseed in enough water to well cover it. Pour off the water. Then infuse the soaked linseed in one pint of water for several hours, standing in a warm place near the fire, stirring occasionally. Then strain off and add four ounces of honey and a handful of raisins. (Will soothe coughs and chest ailments.)

Bran Water. Take two cupfuls of bran and pour over them a quart of tepid water. Allow it to stand overnight. In the morning strain through a cloth, pressing the bran well until all moisture is extracted, and add this water as a base for herb soups, instead of ordinary water.

Herb Soup. Take a quart of bran water, as described above. Then take a cupful each of the following herbs, finely cut: wild mustard tops, chickweed, wild garlic leaves, a few sorrel leaves, and abundant watercress. Pour one pint of water just off the boil on to these herbs, and let them steep for a half-hour. Strain, and then add this to the bran water. Now stir into this mixture one cup of sweet oatmeal, and let all simmer for a few minutes. Thicken with a handful of boiled, peeled and mashed chestnuts. (A truly body-building soup.)

Buttermilk Lemonade. Strain the whey off goat cheese, collecting one pint. Add to this the juice of two small lemons and sweeten with two heaped tablespoons of honey. Serve very cold with a few jasmine (white) flowers added and a handful of blanched almonds. (Andalusia, Spain.)

Medicated Wine. To a pint of sweet red wine add several sprigs of rosemary and wormwood, six candied cherries, two nutmegs, an inch piece of cinnamon bark and candied angelica and bruised root ginger, a dozen large raisins. Allow to steep for one week, keeping in a warm place and shaking every day. Add a further pint of plain, sweet red wine to this, mix well, strain, and take after meals as a blood and nerve tonic.

Strawberry or Cherry Liqueur. Mash ripe strawberries and infuse in sweet, red wine. To every cupful of strawberries add one cupful sugar, two dessertspoons honey, two and a half cupfuls wine. Let the fruit, etc. steep overnight, then strain and chill. Drink this the same day or following day. Place a fresh, whole strawberry in each liqueur glass. Dried cherries (from Turkey and Balkan countries, sold in delicatessen shops by the pound) can be used instead of strawberries to make a delicious drink. Wash the cherries well before use as they are often earthy. The strawberry or cherry residue remaining, after straining off the liqueur, can be used with cream in a trifle sweet.

Brambleberry Wine. Put a quart of blackberries into a pan, cover with boiling water. Stand in a coolish oven over-night to extract the juice. Then strain well into a large stone jar, and ferment (covered) for two weeks. Then add half pound of best cane sugar to every quart of liquid and one dessertspoon of brandy per quart. Seal well. Very good nerve tonic and reviving in feverish colds.

Moorland Tea. Take a handful each of leaves of bilberry, blackberry, speedwell, thyme, wild strawberry, and heather tops. Dry and then mix well. Use as tonic tea, one teaspoon to a cup of water, sweetened with honey. Robert Burns liked this tea.

Cheering Tea. Take a handful each of flower heads of lavender, cornflower, marigold, lime-tree blossom, and a half-handful of flowering sprigs of rosemary and sage, a dessertspoon of dill seeds and a pinch of poppy seeds. Dry the herbs, rubbing the petals free of the flower stalks which should be discarded, and blend with the seeds. Use as common tea, one teaspoon to a cup of water, sweetened with honey. (A remedy against indigestion, headache, fatigue and mental depression. Will aid sound sleep.)

'Hot' Milk. To a pint of bran water (*see* page 192), add one small capsicum pod (cayenne pepper), sliced, a pinch of common pepper, a teaspoon of mustard seed, teaspoon of celery seed, six cloves of cut garlic, a handful of garlic or onion greens. Heat and simmer gently for ten minutes, or until the garlic is soft. Then add one pint of fresh milk, blending slowly. Salt to taste.

193

VARIOUS

Herb Bread. When making wheaten or barley flour bread, add a handful of cooked linseed to the dough, and any of the following aromatic herbs; chives, thyme, chervil, marjoram (or several of these herbs). Chop the herb or herbs finely, and add a heaped tablespoon to every pound of flour. When the dough has risen make a hollow in the centre and add a teaspoon of garlic-flavoured corn oil (garlic cloves steeped for several days in the oil extracted from sweet-corn) to every pound of flour. Allow to rise further and then re-knead to mix in the oil. Brush the tops of the loaves with the garlic-flavoured oil and sprinkle thickly with poppy seeds.

Instead of greasing and flouring the baking tins in the usual way, add a teaspoon of lemon juice to every pound-loaf baking tin, before greasing. This browns the loaves a fine colour and prevents burning. I use lemon juice in all my baking tins (salad oil could replace corn).

Roasted Flour. Sprinkle a half-pound of wheat or barley flour lightly on to a dry baking tin, and place in a warm oven, leaving the door ajar. Shake the tin frequently, and stir and turn over the flour, using a flat knife. Roast the flour until a pale 'biscuit' brown, then set aside to cool. Stir into the flour several teaspoons of roasted poppy seeds or pine kernels, if desired. Can be stored in airtight jars or tins and will keep as well as ordinary biscuits. Eat like a cereal food, with milk, and sweetened with sugar, ground cinnamon or nutmeg, as desired. An excellent food for infants is made by putting a handful of the roasted flour into a basin and mixing into a thin paste with cold milk. Then heat a pint of milk to blood heat and stir this slowly into the cold milk and flour mixture. Sweeten with honey, a little treacle, nutmeg, etc. as liked.

Olives with Herbs. Place a handful of prepared stoned green olives in a pound-size jar, and add the following: three cloves, six pieces of garlic, one sliced cayenne pepper, a sprig of rue, three dried heads of basil flowers, and three large basil leaves, three sprays of dill (green) and rosemary. Fill jar with olive oil.

194

Or half olive oil and half sunflower oil make the herbs taste more strongly. If the olives are for immediate use, several slices of pickled lemon can also be added (the lemon lessens the keeping quality of the olives).

Rose Hips Conserve. Take four pounds of rose hips and a little under two and a half pints cold water. Bring to the boil and simmer for a quarter hour, keeping well stirred. Press the cooked hips through strong muslin for straining. The hips are now ready to make into conserve. To every two pounds of strained hips add one pound of cane sugar and a quarter pound pure honey (not dark honey). Place again in the saucepan, add the juice of half a lemon to every two pounds of the hips-sugar mixture, heat gently and keep well stirred, heating at this low temperature for approximately half an hour (until the jam begins to simmer strongly). Then cook at a faster heat for a further ten minutes. Then remove from the heat and pour into warmed earthen crocks if possible (or into warmed half-pound glass jars — not of larger size). When cooler stir into each jar a half-teaspoon of extract of witch-hazel (as a preservative). When cold, seal with waxed paper. (A blood-cooling conserve. Vitamin and minerals rich.)

A Herbal Tobacco (English gypsy). To a base of dried, finely rubbed coltsfoot leaves, add in smaller proportion (blending to individual taste), thyme, rosemary, eye-bright, ground-ivy and wood-betony, lily-of-the-valley leaves (all or any, as available). All dried and finely sifted. Smoke in a clay pipe.

A Salad to give the Skin a Healthy 'Suntan'. Make a base of watercress, add the leaves of parsley, strawberry, young burdock, and sliced, boiled burdock and salep root. (This recipe is from the writings of the early eleventh-century Arabian herbalist Avicenna who, in his wisdom, noted the effects of herbs — in the diet — upon the human skin.) Salep (Arabic *tha'leb*) was usually in the form of a fine meal ground from the roots of orchidaceous plants.

'A Sallat of floweres.' 'Take of floweres, primrose, cowslip and clove-gilly-floweres, a deep basketful. Cut off their stalkes. Prepare a large glass pot, strew a little sugar in the

bottom, then a layer of floweres, then cover that layer with more sugar, then lay another of the floweres, and then another of the sugar, and this do above one another until the pot be filled to the verie top.

'Then press the floweres and sugar hard down with your hand.

'Then take a sharpe and bitter wine and pour into the pot until it floats above the top layer. Then set in a dry temperature and seal the pot well. Then eat the salat at your pleasure, for it will last fresh until the floweres come again.'

A recipe dedicated to 'the Ladie Frances, Countess Dowager of Exeter, a Seventeenth-centurie Housewife.'

Rosemary. From Bankes Herball. (About seventeenth century.) 'Take the sweet flowres and make powder therof and bynde it to the ryght arme in a lynen clothe and it shall make thee lyght and merrie. Also take the flowres and put them in a chest amonge thy clothes or amonge bookes, and mougthes (moths) shall not hurte them. Also boyle the leves in whyte wyne and wasshe thy face therwith . . . thou shall have a fayre face. Also put the leves under thy beddes heed, and thou shall be delyvered of all evyll dremes. Also take the leves and put them into a vessel of wyne . . . if thou sell that wyne, thou shall have good lucke and spede in the sale. Also make thee a box of the wood and smell it and it shall preserve thy youthe. Also put therof in thy doores or in thy howse and thou shall be withoute dannger of adders and other venymous serpentes. Also make thee a barell therof for the rayne and drynke thou of the drynke that standeth therin and thou nedes to fere no poyson that shall hurte thee. And if thou plante it in thy garden kepe it honestly for it is muche profytable.'

Fertility Herbs. On fertility depends the survival of the human family and the human race. There are many fertility herbs, here are some known to me.

All the mints (except peppermint), basil, balm, marjoram, sage, rosemary, thyme, nasturtium, coriander (including the seed), vervain, bindweed, fumitory, wormwood, southernwood, borage, fennel (including the seed), anise and dill seed, nettle seed, linseed, ginger, cinnamon, cloves, cayenne pepper, liquorice, flowers of red roses and red clover, fruits, juice and tendrils of the grape vine, prepared roots of common purple orchid, raw corn (maize) kernels, raw (flaked) oats, nuts of almond and pistache trees, Summer savory (whole herb), angelica stems, chicory flowers, rue flowers, fennel hearts, heather. The fertility herbs are eaten raw. When palatable mix with salads or cereal flakes. When unpalatable cut small and make into pills, binding them with fine flour and thick honey. General amount of fertility herb is one heaped teaspoon daily (or more if desired) taken until no longer needed.

5

Herbs Applied to Garden and Orchard

Since man first cultivated the earth and planted wild flowers, fruits and vegetables around his home, he began to notice that some plants were protective to others. This phenomenon was explained in many ways before the ecologists took over, and cottage gardeners have applied this knowledge for centuries.

During my travels I have sought out such herbal lore, and wherever I have had a stretch of land for my own use for a while, I have put into practice what I have learnt of this association. In this way, I suppose that I have learnt to treat my plants and trees as I treat my children and animals, feeding tonic herbs to them and surrounding them with the protective ones.

I found that the herbs known as 'aromatics' and 'bitters' were the most important for plant and tree protection. I was not, as I have just said, the first to use such herbs in agriculture. Centuries ago, the Moors were planting rosemary in their fruit gardens to protect their trees and vines from pests. Likewise the French peasants planted onions and garlic and wormwood as protective barriers.

I first discovered by accident the value of the bitter and aromatic herbs as tonics to other plants. This was when I took over an old cottage and apple orchard in the New Forest in England, and there were rats in plenty to eat up my plants as fast as I grew them! So I sprinkled bitter herbs on and around my plants, using such herbs in dry, finely powdered form. This kept the rodents and slugs away and I found that my flowers and vegetables grew to remarkable size as a further result.

This was not quite the first time that I had used one plant to protect another. As long ago as 1947, when I was a gardener to Professor Edmond Bordeux Szekely on his Nature Ranch in Mexico, near the California border, I protected seedlings from the ravages of wild birds, using powdered garlic roots, sprinkled heavily upon and around the seedlings. The idea was a success. The seedlings grew up to safe and healthy maturity, but the garden had a most unpleasant smell after every shower of rain.

Herbs to protect other plants and trees must be either pungently aromatic or extremely bitter. Tomato haulm, after the fruit has been gathered, may be hung on fruit trees, as insect pests do not like its odour. Mexican Indians use tomato haulm in their homes to keep away cockroaches and poisonous insects.

Cayenne pepper is sprinkled on the foliage of fruit trees, before the fruit ripens, to keep away fruit fly. It is a tonic to the tree itself, and harmless to human beings and birds, if any of this pungent, burning pepper-powder should get on to the fruit. But it is disliked by the invading fruit-destroying fly.

Readers of earlier editions of this book have asked me if I know of a complete cure for fruit fly. I do not know and there should NOT be a complete cure, for in my opinion the fruit fly is sent by nature to spoil much of the tree fruits every year, so as to prevent the health of the tree itself being damaged by having to bear unnaturally heavy crops caused by modern cultivation. From my own vines and trees, annually I strip off and throw back to vine or tree almost half of the fruits before they ripen. I have less to sell and eat, but quality of fruit is better and the trees keep strong and healthy.

Aromatic bitters such as wormwood, southernwood, mugwort, rue and others mentioned in this book as insect repellents, also deter birds at seed-planting times. Beans, peas, ground-nuts, and the grains of cereals, and all other types of seed which birds like to eat, are sprinked with such herbs (dried and finely powdered). I myself sprinkle the seeds themselves *as I plant them in the soil*, before I put the top-soil over them. This protecting powder also deters rats and mice and other seed-stealing creatures. I and many other gardeners in many parts of the world, using this herbal treatment, have had no failures in growing maximum crops. These dried herbs are also a tonic to the seeds which they are protecting. French peasants plant scillas to deter moles.

It is possible to utilize the absorptive properties of sphagnum moss in plant protection. A strong brew is made from the already mentioned bitter herbs, and the dried sphagnum is saturated in this. The saturated moss is then packed around the plants and will retain its protective power even during heavy rain and strong winds which would wash or blow away herbal dusts.

As insect repellents (plants of old-time use by gardeners and farmers) such things as the powdered heads of African Daisy, *pyrethrum*, powdered Derris root, and tobacco dust, are still in great demand. The much acclaimed chemical and poisonous products, which have done such vast and as yet unestimated damage to the health of human beings, animals, birds and bees as well as to the crops and trees on which they have been used, have lost much of their former popularity. Nor are the poisonous chemical sprays very effective. For instance I have noted many times that people living in houses screened against mosquitoes, and at the same time using chemical poison sprays (once mostly containing D.D.T.) against such mosquitoes as do manage to enter their dwellings despite the screening, are more troubled with mosquito bites than my family who sleep out-of-doors when living in hot climates, without any netting or screening against mosquitoes, and merely relying on a lotion of herbs applied to faces and hands. We are rarely bitten, even when we have been living in such mosquito-infested areas as the coconut groves of tropical Mexico, or the marshes of the French Carmargue.

There are herbs available for disinfecting the soil. The best of these, and the easiest to grow, are mustard and sage. Mustard grows very rapidly and is a cheap crop. At flowering-time it is cut and dug into the ground. It is a tonic to other plants and kills off the eggs of insects which may be in the soil. Such use of mustard is not new; it is advocated in old farming journals and books, especially around the time of Queen Victoria, before the great swing-over to chemical fertilizers and soil treatments. Sage is new to me. I have never found this use of it advised in any old agricultural books (which I used to study once with the same enthusiasm that many of my friends have for detective stories). I learnt its use from Professor Szekely in Mexico, and he in turn learnt it from the Mexican Indian workers on his lands where he grows thousands of acres of grapes.

Sage drops its leaves very prolifically twice a year, and they are swept up and mixed with goat manure and wood-ash and then given to other plants, especially vines and corn; and what superb crops result! When American agricultural inspectors saw Professor Szekely's wonderful grapes, and were informed that he never used chemical sprays or fertilizers in his vine-yards, and gave his vines scarcely any water, the inspectors refused to accept such *natural* treatment of vines! They declared that the professor's workers must be buying both chemical sprays and fertilizers themselves and using them without telling him!

Since my Mexican days I have recently, in the hills of Upper Galilee, using the same Mexican method, and with an abundance of wild sage plants at my disposal, grown wonderful grapes. Within two years of beginning the work I had the biggest vines in the village, although the vines on other land in the village were many years older. The agricultural authorities of the region have praised this successful use of sage as a plant tonic.

Grow comfrey in the garden. For as well as supplying leaves of the utmost medicinal value for man and animals, comfrey plants are beneficial to other plants. Being deep-rooting, they do not take away the minerals in the surface soil from other plants growing close to them, and they keep the surrounding soil rich and moist and give protective shade and shelter to other plants, with their large, rough leaves. I find my comfrey plants (the roots imported from England by post) of great help in Israel: not only for the salad herb that their young leaves provide, and the medicine of the older leaves, but also on account of the parasol shade that this plant gives to my seedlings under the fierce sun of Israel in spring and summertime.

Wood-ash is not exactly a herb; but it is made from vegetable matter. As a fine powder it is a wonderful plant food, excellent for fruit trees. Daily in winter-time I make wood fires, and I save every ounce of the ash with as much care as if it were pure gold dust; it is almost of like value in my estimation. Sprinkled on pea and bean pods, tomatoes and soft fruits, it deters birds and rodents, does not leave an unpleasant taste and can be washed off easily. Also it is harmless to plant and to man.

Powdered charcoal sprinked on root vegetables is an excellent preventative of insect pests, wire worms, etc., and so is straw burnt on the soil surface before sowing fragile seeds such as onion and many varieties of lettuce. A mere sprinkle per plant, more for trees, provides extra minerals, deters root pests, conserves moisture.

Every year I discard my old stores of dried herbs and replace with new season herbs. The old, I scatter around plants.

The result of the use of these recommended things of Nature in the growing of plants and trees, is wonderful crops, flowers of great size, bright colouring and rich scents, vegetables and fruits which are healthy, good-tasting and long-keeping (for instance harvested my grapes will remain in perfect condition for weeks in a midsummer in Israel, whereas shop-bought grapes, heavily irrigated, chemical-sprayed, and given chemical fertilizers in the growing of them, turn bad overnight).

Experts such as J. L. Chase, founder of the agricultural firm of Chase Ltd., and agricultural inspectors in Israel, have seen and praised the crops grown and protected with the aid of herbs.

I have noted that ants dislike the pungency of herbal dusts, and I have removed ant-hills from my flower-beds merely by using on them my stale aromatic herbs (mixed with wood-ash), when changing my herbal supplies for the new ones of each season.

Arab and Yemenite farmers in Israel proclaim proudly that they do not use chemical sprays or fertilizers on their crops. Some of them do make use of chemicals, but most of them do not. I noticed recently when a party of Yemenite farmers were taking over land for crops, that they brought along their sacks of wood-ash for the improvement of the soil. They use *habba* (basil) as insecticide.

It is in Israel that I have found a use for the thorns and thistles which were created as a curse on the land (Genesis iii. 18). Thistles and some of the very spiky thorns such as 'dom' and bramble, and also the plant sea-holly, cut when green, and banked around the feet of fruit trees, especially peach and almond trees which are much eaten by pests, will receive ample protection from the creeping pests such as caterpillars and grubs, which hatch out in the ground and then climb up into the trees. It is especially important to cut the thistles when green, for then their prickles are placed very close together. As they get older the stems lengthen and the prickles become wider apart, leaving uncovered stems to make bridges across the barricade, along which the invaders could travel. The difference to be seen between protected and unprotected trees is very impressive. And the spiky barricade does not harm the trees in any way and can be removed in the winter-time, when the trees are sleeping and have nothing to offer pests. I use thorny brush to keep birds from bush fruits, and with the same idea I allow brambles to grow up around my vines, they protect from 'snatch and run' thieving by man as well as by birds!

Thorny branches thrust down mole holes discourage their over populous presence in gardens and orchards (as does the growing of wormwood, southernwood and rue).

It is notable that soft-bodied predators such as slugs and snails do not like the roughness of common 'brake' (bracken), so this makes a better litter for strawberries than straw.

The seaweed group of plants (Algae), green or brown or red, and including bladder-wrack, sea-wracks generally, sea-lettuce, carrageen, provides a most valuable organic fertilizer for cultivated land on garden or field scale. The seaweeds may be used either well-rotted or dried and finely powdered. Generally speaking, about a handful is required per plant per year, with a half bucket per year for trees larger than saplings, and for these the application must be proportionate to size.

When packing plants for the market (either cut or with roots) dampened sphagnum moss packed around them is a great help to keep them well.

Finally, because this is a chapter about Nature Gardening with herbs, although the following is not really about using herbs but on growing them, I am writing about the influence of the moon on crops at their planting-time.

This 'moon-planting' is not new, is indeed very old. The Moors centuries ago were experts on this planting rhythm, having studied very carefully the influences of the moon on crops.

The following is from an old manuscript, later printed at the Unicorn Press in Paternoster Row, London (in 1631), the precepts of which I have carefully followed over many years.

'These plants can be sown at all times of the moon: spinach, parsnip, carrot, radish, lettuce. In the new of the moon and early in the year, sow the pot herbes such as marjoram, thyme, basil, etc. rosemary and lavender, and most flowers, especially white poppy, double marigolds, sweet rocket, gilliflowers, and sow the gourds, including cucumber and melons in the full of the moon. Sow parsley, aniseed, dill, etc., mints, violets and pansies. Old moon, onions, leeks, cabbage and all the brassicas. In the gathering of seed for the next season sowings, only gather at the wane of the moon and in fine, dry, weather.'

That the moon has extraordinary influence even on the smallest organisms is shown in the power of the moon on such tiny things as thread-worms embedded in the intestines of a child or animal. The worms are far more active when the moon is full (as are all kinds of worms), and herbalists know that that is the best time to dose worm-infested creatures, in order to expel the worms. But nowadays the human race have shut out moonlight from their lives almost entirely. Only the nomad people now sleep out beneath the moon. Moonlight is needed for whole health and fertility of all creatures (stabled animals likewise suffer from this deprivation) and that is why I favour sleeping outdoors, and when sleeping indoors is necessary, then at least windows should be kept open and uncurtained.

Indoor plants should be put out into the moonlight and starlight just as they should enjoy sunlight for total health.

I worked out in this matter of moon planting, that things for which strong roots are required should be planted when the moon is waning — for example, vine and berry cuttings, and the legumes. Where strong upper growth is desired — for example, all cereals, most vegetables, etc. — plant when the moon is waxing middle or full. Plant roses and perennials when mid-waxing.

Alberico Boncompagni Ludovisi (the Prince of Venosa, Italy), a dedicated nature farmer, has for many years successfully followed my moon planting method for his vines and cereal crops on his lands outside Rome.

6

Conclusion

Johann von Cube wrote in his *Herbal*, printed in the year 1485 — 'I thank thee, O Creator of heaven and earth, who has given powers to the plants and other created things contained in this book, that thou hast granted me the grace to reveal this treasure, which until now has lain buried and hid from the sight of common men.'

I do not make such high claims for my herbal. But, far and constant travels during the past thirty years, and my life shared mostly with peasants of Spain, gypsies of Spain and many other lands from Turkey to North America, Mexican Indians, Berber and Bedouin Arabs, and others, all of them natural herbalists, have given me opportunities to collect first-hand knowledge much of which I do not think can be found in earlier herbals.

Of course not all of this book is original by any means. Herbalists share their common remedies, just as the orthodox doctors have their common chemical and vaccine treatments, all universal.

These people whom I have mentioned, the peasants, the gypsies, the Arabs and others, shared their herbal knowledge with me because they sensed my instinctive faith in this form of medicine, which really grew from my love of the wild plants of the world, with me from early childhood. (I always wanted to be a jobbing gardener by profession, but my father would not permit this; he allowed me to study veterinary medicine instead, because from early days I had skill with animals.)

For my part, I exchanged with my primitive herbal teachers new cures — new to them — which I had learnt in other lands. Sometimes I was able to cure my teachers, members of their family, or their animals, of ailments which had not yielded to their own remedies because they did not know of the more effective herbs for those particular ills.

However, out of this carefully and slowly collected herbal knowledge, I know, as other herbalists before me have known, that there is no wonder herb able to cure all the ills of mankind.

Herbs have great powers (which no chemist can excel or even imitate fully), as can be shown by countless examples. For instance the purging effect of a few senna pods steeped in cold water, the effect of the male-fern root upon a tapeworm hooked to the intestines of a human body, the soothing effect of raw cucumber juice on inflamed eyes, or of rue leaves applied to stings of poisonous insects, or of sage tea to relieve a bad cough — and all the other examples of herbal treatments to be found in this book, each one of them powerful.

But in the treatment of disease, other means are usually needed to help the herbs to do their curative work. Sick people need to cleanse themselves through short fasts on herbal teas and fruit juices and to take herbal laxatives, or they should semi-fast on fruits and fresh milk. They also need fresh air, ample sleep and mental tranquility for a complete cure of any kind of ailment, be it a broken limb or a fever. Also faith is needed to persevere with herbal treatments which are sometimes very slow in their curative action, and which sometimes are seen to worsen the symptoms of the ailment before curing it. Moreover, certain beneficial effects can be misinterpreted as disasters (*see*, for example, Strawberry rash, mentioned on page 158).

'Fast and pray,' said Christ, one of the greatest healers in the history of the world. A good example of the slowness of herbs, and of lack of faith in those using them, was given some years ago after World War II, in an article published in the *News Chronicle*. The article appealed to me because it told of a gypsy herbalist and her use of one of the herbs which I love best, elder blossom. It concerned a soldier blinded at Dunkirk and considered incurable. A travelling gypsy woman saw the blind soldier and noted his sadness; she advised the use of elder blossom as a treatment for the eyes.

The soldier's father carefully applied the treatment: the elder blossom began to cause pain in the soldier's eyes, and the family lost faith and stopped the treatment. But on a further visit the gypsy met the soldier again and saw that his eyes had improved. She persuaded the family to continue with the elder blossom, and the final result was that full sight was restored to the soldier's eyes. (One day, in his world of darkness, he saw a glimmer. It was his mother's wedding ring. Slowly the power of sight returned to the blind eyes.) It would be cruel and misleading to assert that this outcome of the treatment was inevitable: but it is certainly worth trying.

Often when following or giving herbal treatments, cure has seemed hopeless. But I have had faith, telling myself that the particular herb must cure; it has always cured that specific ailment through the ages: it was put on earth to cure such an ailment, and the knowledge of its use was given to mankind by God who created the medicinal plants.

Chemicals do not mix well with herbs. Use one treatment or the other, but do not try to use both at once.

Professor Edmond Szekely of Hungary, who has achieved many wonderful herbal cures with people whom chemical drug treatments could not cure (I have met many of his cases, restored to excellent health) has discussed in his books, and has described to me personally, the lasting harm frequently caused by chemical drugs and substances of modern sera treatments, which, being unnatural to the human body, have lodged in various organs and defied removal. He declares that it is often more difficult to cure a person of the drugs taken when ill than to cure the illness itself.

CONCLUSION

In the Materia Medica chapter of this book I mention some of the plants which herbalists of many lands have found beneficial in the treatment of cancer. Cures appear to have been achieved with some of them, especially with red clover flowers, violet leaves and flowers, and vine leaves. However, I consider that although these cancer-treatment herbs may give much relief and retard the growth of cancer, a complete cure is very unlikely, once the human body has degenerated in health sufficiently for such a destructive illness as cancer to grow within it. It is wiser to plan a daily personal campaign against cancer, by cultivating a happy and contented mind, breathing unpolluted air, drinking clean water (free from unnatural additions of chemicals), eating natural foods (and in their raw form as much as possible), making use of Nature's abundant herbs, and taking sufficient physical exercise (for without ample exercise total health is not possible).

I consider that herbs are a sacred medicine, promised to man in the Bible. The mystics and the great healers such as that ancient Jewish sect, the Essenes, of which many say that Christ was a member, were herbalists.

I am thankful that right through the ages (discounting the misuse of herbs in Black Magic) herbs have been kept a 'clean' medicine. There has been no association with experiments on laboratory animals — sentient creatures loving life as the normal human being loves life, and yet deprived by man of all their right to a natural life, and made artificially diseased, degraded and then killed, usually without any thought of shame or regret in the deed from the killer.

I like the observation from Dr. Cameron Gruner, M.D., in his book *The Canon of Medicine of Avicenna*:

'Watching the medicinal trees and shrubs and herbs in this way: seeing their properties by their forms and colours and odours, and their changes in character with the changes of the seasons, and alternation of drought and plenty — how great is the wonder of the work of Nature! We note how substances are being elaborated into plants, which we, wanting their help, know how to take at the crucial moment: "Now we must draw the resin, now we must take these flowering tops", and so on. But we are not the only watchers. The bees have been waiting, and the birds, and the slugs, the ants, the herbivora — all these and many others waiting to draw from such supplies that which is applicable to their requirements. Nature herself also waits for these to be collected from her treasury. It is for us ourselves not to pass them by. If we did nothing more than study the Materia Medica of ancient days we should have ample material for thought, and become cognisant of the link between that age and this. The herbs are still cultivated and still used in the East in the manner of the past.'

I have learnt much herbal medicine from the wild creatures, noting the herbs that they select for their food or medicine. I have taken note of the desire of all wild animals for the fresh garlics and clovers as well as their dislike of these when plucked and withered and used as plant protectors; the love of birds for chickweed and rose hips, of the tortoise for sorrel and dandelion, of the rabbits and hares for milk-thistle and bramble leaves, of the foxes and snakes for the vines, of the bears for the blueberry plants (bilberries); an endless list. And the bees! With their exceptional instinct they are seekers of the most medicinal of the herbs. The bees will pass by large flowers rich in easily obtainable, available nectar, and choose instead the tiny flowerlets of lavender or sage, rosemary or balm (the bees share my own love for the aromatics, many of which are in the Labiatae family, one that is very rich in medicinal properties).

I would rather prescribe for animals than humans, because at least in our modern world, animals are usually healthier (except, of course, the caged ones). So many of us are to some extent mentally ill: sadness or rage or fear will retard much of the healing work of the herbs, and that is why I try to insist on what is present-day wellnigh unattainable — a tranquil spirit.

When my publishers asked me to write this herbal book for human use, in place of my usual veterinary herbal writings, my first thought was to refuse, because I was worried that readers of such a herbal might write to me for individual medical advice and prescriptions. I could never find the time to be involved in such correspondence. In any case I am constantly travelling, most letters sent to me never reach me, and those that do come into my hands are frequently lost because I have not the time in which to answer them. They are put on one side and remain a worry at the back of my mind, while I try to make time to attend to them as well as all my crowding daily tasks. In addition to the usual care of a home, with teenage children claiming much attention, I have my trees and plants, my herbs and bees, and usually many animals. There is my daily herbal work, consuming so many hours; the growing of the herbs; their collecting and drying and storing and making up into preparations for various requirements. I am enthusiastic about the maintenance of good health through natural methods, yet I sometimes think that my habitual lack of sleep, because my days are too short to manage all the pressing work, will eventually destroy me. This I must write here, for it is not easy to make people understand what a burden letter-writing can be.

If readers will study this herbal, if this form of medicine really appeals to them as it has always appealed to me, they will become herbalists themselves. For this reason, because I cannot offer individual help, I have given much care to making the dosage of the herbs sufficiently clear for readers to follow without difficulty: I hope I have succeeded in this. On pages 27 and 28 I have listed a few names of suppliers of herbs and herbal products.

I wish for all readers of this herbal book the health and happiness that herbs have given to my children and myself.

I quote again from the Bible; of Ahab's longing for a herb garden: 'And Ahab spake unto Naboth, saying, "Give me thy vineyard that I may have it for a garden of herbs, because it is near unto my house".'

Every family with a bit of land should plant a herb garden. It will bring them closer to Nature, and that is always a good thing for Everyman.

And for those who are compelled to live in apartments with no land available at all, there is always the plant pot and the window-box (that is if the city air is pure enough and not entirely fouled with fumes from crowding vehicles or nearby factories). Remember to use charcoal and rubble as foundation for the pots and boxes and to feed the plants with the same care as one's own children. Such as providing the plants with some fresh topsoil every week and taking precautions not to over-water, but to wash the foliage free from city grime frequently, though not doing so during sunlight or in cold spells. Collect rainwater for the plants, and arrange their placing so that they get sunlight.

Suitable plants for such cultivation are basil, chives, marjoram, dwarf rosemary, geraniums (including the scented verbena-rose), mints, sorrel, parsley, borage, and the annuals; mustard and cress, coriander, dill, nasturtium, marigold, sweet-peas, larkspur, and many more.

Finally, love your plants, your land; only then will all truly flourish. I have loved mine always and that is why they have grown so wonderfully everywhere, for on my travels I have made many gardens and vineyards.

Good growing!

A NOTE FROM THE AUTHOR

I sincerely regret that it is no longer possible to answer readers' problems sent to me in the post. Because I travel so much, months often go by without mail reaching me and very many letters are lost.

Furthermore, my herbal books are published in many foreign translations, in addition to the British and American editions, and if all those countless thousands who now have my books were to write to me for personal advice, my every day and most of every night would be fully taken in writing letters. Impossible! Nor can I, in fairness, answer a few chosen persons and not answer all. Unjust. Again impossible! Therefore no longer can I answer readers' letters.

Indexes

GENERAL INDEX WITH NAMES OF HERBS AND RECIPES
FOR HERBAL TREATMENTS (See separate index for *Disorders and
diseases amenable to herbal treatment*)

213

Index

Milkwort, 113
Mint: 113–14; tea, 113, 114
Mistletoe, 114
Moles, 48, 200, 203
Moon's influence on growth, crops, 204–5
Moorland Tea, 193
'Mortification Plant', see Mallow
Mullein, 114–15
Mustard, as soil cleanser, 201
Mustard, Black, 115–16

Natural Rearing products, 28
Nasturtium, 116–17
Nettle, 117–18; Dead (White) Nettle, 118; cooked nettles, 117
Nut Galls, against toothache, 187

Oak Moss (Lungs of Oak), 185, 187
Oatmeal Gruel, 191–2
Oats, 118–19
Old Man's Beard, see Virgin's Bower
Olives with Herbs, 194–5
Onion: as poultice, 26; planted as protective barrier, 198
Opium poppy, 119–20
Orchards, use of herbs in, 198–204
Orchis, 120–2
Orris Root, 99
Our Lady's Milk Thistle, see Holy Thistle

Paeon, ancient Greek herbalist, 124
Pansy, 122
Paracelsus, Male Fern praised by, 74
Parsley, 122–3
Parsnip, wild, 123–4; to serve, 124
Pennyroyal, 124
Peony, 124–5
Peppermint, 125–6
Periwinkle, 126
Peruvian bark, in toothpaste, 183
Pilewort, see Celandine, Lesser
Pillows, herbal, see Mignonette, Sweet Cecily
Pills, Herbal, home-made, 27
Pimpernel, 126
Plantain, 127–8
Pliny, Male Fern praised by, 74
'Poor Man's Bread', see Watercress

Poppy, see Opium poppy; Poppy-head poultice, 26
Poppy, Red Field, 128–9
Pot-pourri (Provençal), 184–5
Preparing herbs, 21–8
Preserving herbs, 18–21; by quick-freezing, 21
Primrose, 129
Puffball, 129
Pumpkin, 129–30
Purslane, 130–2

Queen of Hungary's Water, 139, 184
'Queen of the Meadow', 132–3
Quince, 133–4
Quinsy Berry, see Currant, Black

Ragwort, 134
Raspberry, 134–5; see also Blackberry
Recipes, various, 182–6, 190–7
Red Currant, 65–6
Reed, 135–6
Remedies to prepare, 186–90
Rhubarb, Wild, 136
Rock Rose, 137
Roman Pill Nettle, 117
Rose, Briar, 137
Rose Hips Conserve, 195
Rosemary, 138–40; remedy for colds from, 186
Royal Fern, 75–6; Jelly, 75
Rubbing Lotion, to make, 188
Rue, 140–2; against stings and bites, 189
Rye-grass, 142

Safflower, 142–4
Sage, 144–5; against bites and stings, 189; in gargle, 186; as hair tonic, 183–4; for cleaning teeth, 182–3; Sage Tea, 144–5; uses of, in garden (leaves, etc.), 201
St. John's Girdle, see Wormwood
St. John's Wort, 145–6; Crusaders' use of, 145; for poultice bandage, 26–7
Salad Burnet, 42
'Salad for Suntan', 195
Salep, 195; see Orchis
'Sallat of Flowers', 195–6

216

Index

INDEX OF DISORDERS AND DISEASES AMENABLE TO HERBAL TREATMENTS, WITH PRINCIPAL RECOMMENDATIONS